MADE TO
CRAVE
Devotional

Also by Lysa TerKeurst

MADE TO CRAVE

Devotional

60 Days TO CRAVING GOD, NOT FOOD

LYSA TERKEURST

New York Times **Bestselling Author**

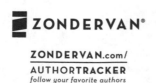

ZONDERVAN®

ZONDERVAN.com/
AUTHORTRACKER
follow your favorite authors

ZONDERVAN

Made to Crave Devotional
Copyright © 2011 by Lysa TerKeurst

This title is also available as a Zondervan ebook. Visit www.zondervan.com/ebooks.

This title is also available in a Zondervan audio edition. Visit www.zondervan.fm.

Requests for information should be addressed to:

Zondervan, *Grand Rapids, Michigan* 49530

Library of Congress Cataloging-in-Publication Data

TerKeurst, Lysa.
      Made to crave devotional : 60 days to craving God, not food / Lysa TerKeurst.
        p. cm.
      ISBN 978-0-310-33470-5 (softcover)
       1. Christian women—Religious life. 2. Devotional literature. 3. God
(Christianity)—Worship and love. 4. Spirituality. 5. Food—Religious
aspects—Christianity. I. Title.
      BV4527.T46252 2011
      242'.643—dc23   2011040630

Published in association with the literary agency of Fedd & Company, Inc., Post Office Box 341973, Austin, TX 78734.

Cover design: Curt Diepenhorst
Cover photography: Getty Image®
Interior design: Beth Shagene

Printed in the United States of America

18 19 20 21 /LSC/ 28 27 26 25 24 23 22

Contents

A Personal Word for You

I know how vulnerable this issue of healthy eating can be. I wrote about the tender and tortured details of my own food battles in the book, *Made to Crave: Satisfying Your Deepest Desire with God, Not Food*. In it, I shared what the Bible has to say about why we put ourselves through all the hard work it takes to lose weight only to regain it and then find ourselves stuck in a vicious cycle. It wasn't an easy topic for me to write about, and I second-guessed myself more than once. But when the book was published, I was overwhelmed by the response. I heard from thousands of women who not only identified with my struggles, but who were also finding victory in their efforts to eat healthier.

Many readers told me that the book got them off to a great start, but they wanted even more guidance and encouragement to help them stay motivated and on track. That's why I wrote the *Made to Crave Devotional*. It's packed with sixty inspirational entries to give you a daily power boost of encouragement. There is plenty of new material here that isn't in the original book, but rest assured that I've also included readers' favorite nuggets of wisdom from *Made to Crave*.

Just like the *Made to Crave* book, this devotional is not a how-to-get-healthy book. One look at the diet shelf in any bookstore and you'll know there are already plenty of how-to books to choose from. And the authors of those books all appear to have cravings for carrot sticks, not to mention abs of steel (and buns that have never sagged or tummies that have never tried to pop out over the tops of their jeans).

I, on the other hand, know what less athletic women crave. And I am well acquainted with the words *muffin top* and *cellulite*. Muffin tops and cellulite with stretch marks, thank you very much and have a nice day. I also know what it's like to feel sad and powerless in this battle to get healthy.

I want to lead Jesus girls on a journey that will help them find a stick-to-itiveness and a lasting want-to that taps into something much more powerful than the surface desires of wanting to weigh less and wear a smaller size. We need to tap into this power because the battle we face isn't just with sugary, fatty, or salty foods. There is a spiritual battle going on. It's real. And it's amazing how perfectly the Bible gives us specific ways to find victory with our food struggles.

Even for girls like us who don't crave carrot sticks.

Lysa TerKeurst

Unsettled

*The Son is the radiance of God's glory and the exact
representation of his being, sustaining all things by his powerful
word. After he had provided purification for sins,
he sat down at the right hand of the Majesty in heaven.*
(HEBREWS 1:3)

Thought for the Day: Unsettle me in the best kind of way. For when
I allow your touch to reach the deepest parts of me — dark and dingy
and hidden away too long — suddenly, a fresh wind of life twists and
twirls and dances through my soul.

The year I finally got my eating issues under control, I started with
a very simple New Year's prayer. I didn't write a long list of resolu-
tions as I had in previous years. After all, my list from one year to
the next could have simply been a photocopy from the year before.
It was the same stuff, year after year. I started out with great gusto
to eat less, move more, make this a healthy lifestyle, and live in victory. Yadda, yadda, yadda.

But each year around January 7, I'd get invited to a party where treats were plentiful and motivation scarce. My stomach would soon be overstuffed and my resolve worn quite thin.

Year after year.

But this year I just couldn't bring myself to write the list again. So, I prayed this simple prayer: *Unsettle me.*

These are the words I wrote in my journal …

Unsettle me. These are the two words rattling about in my brain today. I almost wish it were a more glamorous prayer. Surely more eloquent words could be found for what I'm feeling led to pursue during this New Year. But these are the words, this is the prayer for my 2009.

The funny thing is, I've spent my whole existence trying to find a place to settle down, people to settle down with, and a spirit about me worthy of all this settled down-ness. All of this is good. A contented heart, thankful for its blessings, is a good way to settle.

But there are areas of my life that have also settled that mock my desires to be a godly woman — compromises, if you will. Attitudes that I've wrapped in the lie, "Well, that's just how I am. And if that's all the bad that's in me, I'm doing pretty good."

I dare you, dear soul of mine, to notice the stark evidence of a spirit that is tainted and a heart that must be placed under the microscope of God's Word. Yes, indeed, unsettle me, Lord.

Unearth that remnant of justification.

Shake loose that pull toward compromise.

Reveal that broken shard of secrecy.

Expose that tendency to give up.

Unsettle me in the best kind of way. For when I allow Your touch to reach the deepest parts of me — dark and dingy and hidden away too long—suddenly, a fresh wind of life twists and twirls and dances through my soul.

I can delight in hope that this is my year to change.

I can discover reasons to appreciate my body and find softer ways for my thoughts to land.

I can recognize the beauty of discipline and crave the intimacy with God it unleashes.

I can rest assured though the journey will be hard, I will be held.

Goodbye to my remnants, my justification, shards, and tendencies. This is not who I am—nor who I was created to be.

Goodbye to shallow efforts, self-focus, and suspicious fears that I'll never find victory in this area of my life. I am an unsettled woman who no longer wishes to take part in distractions or destructions.

Welcome deeper love for God and the realization I am made for more than this constant battle. Welcome my unsettled heart.

Are you ready to be unsettled in a good way?

Maybe you are at the beginning of your journey and feel intimidated by the long road ahead. Or, maybe you are on the other end of the spectrum and need ongoing encouragement to stay healthy. Whether you're in those places or somewhere in the middle, will you make a renewed commitment now? Will you ask God to unsettle you in the midst of where you are? And then dare to keep turning these pages and holding tight to God's transforming truth.

Dear Lord, make me a courageous woman who isn't
afraid to pray this prayer over and over in the days ahead.
In Jesus' name. Amen.

What If I Let God Down?

Do not fear, for I am with you; do not be dismayed,
for I am your God. I will strengthen you and help you;
I will uphold you with my righteous right hand.

(ISAIAH 41:10)

Thought for the Day: I wept as I realized this would be one of the most significant spiritual journeys of my life. A spiritual journey that would yield great physical benefits.

I recently received an email from a woman who wrote, "Lysa, one of my greatest fears in reading *Made to Crave* is not just letting myself down, but even worse, letting God down."

I understand how she feels. When you've tried and failed as many times as I have, you start to feel gun-shy about trying again. I'd lose the weight, feel great for a couple of months, deceive myself into thinking I could return to old habits, and all the weight would creep back on. I'd failed at finding lasting victory with every other attempt, even with programs I thought were the sure thing. So, why would this one be any different?

And why in heavens would I want to add spiritual guilt on top of my physical guilt? Why would I risk the shame of making God look bad too?

Guilt wrapped in shame is a terrible burden to carry. Guilt always came when I knew I was making poor choices and could see the scale numbers climbing. Shame came when my weight gain became apparent to everyone else in the world. Battling something so raw, so deeply personal was hard; knowing my failures were apparent to everyone else added humiliation to my toxic stew of emotions.

Yes, the physical struggle was hard enough. I certainly didn't want to drag down my spiritual life with this struggle as well.

But here's the problem: whether or not I wanted to admit it, my weight issues were already dragging me down spiritually. When I don't have peace physically, I don't have peace spiritually. I can't separate the two. Nor should I. I need spiritual motivation to step in where my physical determination falls short. *that's good!*

So I started reading the Bible from the perspective of someone struggling with food issues. Though I had read the Bible many times and have even taught Bible studies for years, I'd missed how much God cares about and talks about this issue. Tucked within this book written thousands of years ago are some of the most astounding and life-changing truths directly applicable to this modern-day unhealthy eating epidemic that plagues women.

I wept with joy. I wept with relief. I wept as I realized this would be one of the most significant spiritual journeys of my life. A spiritual journey that would yield great physical benefits. And what about my concerns with letting God down?

My pastor, Steven Furtick, put that to rest one day with a simple but very profound truth, "How can you let God down when you weren't ever holding Him up?"

I had to choose to operate in the reassurance of God's love, the remembrance of God's grace, and the reality of God's power. And, according to Isaiah 41:10, God is the one holding me up, not the other way around. To that I say, "Amen!"

Dear Lord, this is one of the most significant spiritual journeys of my life. Help me to focus on You as I battle this raw, personal issue. I need You today. In Jesus' name. Amen.

Yes Jesus!
I always need
You!
7-19-18

The Right Questions

Peter and the other apostles replied:
"We must obey God rather than human beings!"
(ACTS 5:29)

Thought for the Day:
I must obey God rather than the scale!

My friend, Karen Ehman, was a great cheerleader during my healthy eating journey. On one of her "Weight Loss Wednesday" blog posts she wrote something I found incredibly insightful.* The biggest shift in her motivation from her yo-yo dieting days was replacing the delight of diminishing numbers on the scale with the delight of obedience to God.

Karen wrote:

I was very hopeful as I hopped on the scale this morning. I kept track of my food, exercised five days at the gym for 30–45 minutes, and my jeans were zipping up much easier than expected.

---

*You can connect with Karen and read all her great Weight Loss Wednesday's posts at www.KarenEhman.com.

So, I whipped the scale out ... and I'd lost a measly 1.8 pounds! What!?! I was sure it would say at least two or maybe even three. I felt gypped. And I felt like running to the kitchen to make a frozen waffle or two so I could slather it with real butter, spread it with some Peter Pan, and douse it with a load of pure maple syrup to stick it to that scale! Then I stopped and remembered what I felt the Lord saying this week.

Define your week by obedience, not by a number on the scale.

The scale does help measure our progress, but it can't tell us everything. It can't tell us if too much salt intake is making us retain a pound or two of water. It can't tell us if we actually lost a pound of fat, but gained more muscle from weight training. And, it can't tell us what time of the month it is and give us automatic credit for the extra two pounds or so that those glorious few days bring to us.

So, I had to stop and ask myself the following questions:

- Did I overeat this week on any day? No.
- Did I move more and exercise regularly? Yes.
- Did I eat in secret or out of anger or frustration? No.
- Did I feel that, at any time, I ran to food instead of to God? Nope.
- Before I hopped on the scale, did I think I'd had a successful, God-pleasing week? Yep!

So, why oh why do I get so tied up in a stupid number? And why did I almost let it trip me up and send me to the kitchen for a 750-calorie binge? Don't worry. I had a yogurt and tea instead.

Sweet friends, we need to define ourselves by our obedience, not a number on the scale. We are all in this thing together. And we will get the weight off, even if it is 1.8 pounds at a time!

I love what Karen says about defining ourselves by our obedience and not by a number on the scale—or, for me, what size my clothes are or how I feel seeing models with unattainable sizes on the magazine covers.

Yes, eating healthy and exercising gets our bodies into better shape, but we are never supposed to get soul satisfaction from our looks. Our looks are temporary; if we hitch our souls to this fleeting pursuit, we'll quickly become disillusioned. The apostle Paul wrote, "We must obey God rather than human beings" (Acts 5:29). I read that verse differently now: "I must obey God rather than human values—like a number on the scale or the size on the tag in my jeans." The only true satisfaction we can seek is the satisfaction of being obedient to the Lord.

Dear Lord, I don't want to define myself by a number on my scale or any other human value. I truly want to be obedient to You each day. Help me to follow hard after You. In Jesus' name. Amen.

Consider It

Consider it pure joy, my brothers and sisters,
whenever you face trials of many kinds.
(JAMES 1:2)

Thought for the Day:
Triumph in this choice will produce a blessing.

This verse can be hard to swallow. When tears are plentiful and answers are few, it's hard to be joyful. And though I know there are many more serious trials than my weight struggles, issues in this area make me feel vulnerable, incapable, and insecure. Not joyful.

I find it hard to "consider it pure joy." However, one reason the phrase "consider it" starts off this teaching in James is because we will probably not *feel* it. In the midst of a trial, we will probably not *feel* the joy, the hope, or the encouragement tucked within this verse—we have to *consider* it.

On your healthy eating journey there will be times when you face trials. You may not have considered them trials in the past. But when you're tempted to stray from the commitment to make healthier choices, it's a trial.

Perhaps you, like me, have faced this scenario. You enter a restaurant enthused with your plan to order the tropical salad with grilled chicken. You actually like this yummy salad and know that you will be satisfied with this healthy dish. But then the juiciest, most tempting bacon cheeseburger with a large side of French fries presents itself as an option. Of course, it's the feature photo on the menu and a platter is being delivered to the next table just before the server comes to take your order. I know, we've all been there —this is a trial.

We had decided ahead of time on a satisfying salad. But in a moment of weakness, the justifications for a burger and fries start rolling around in our minds.

Certainly moderation is good. And had we budgeted for a burger that day, so be it. But if we decided ahead of time that a salad would be the satisfying choice, we'd do well to stick with what we'd decided before the moment of temptation.

It's so easy to slip into an all-out reversal of all our progress, so we have to be careful. Remember, our ultimate goal is peace — physically, emotionally, and spiritually. If this meal choice threatens to send us into a tailspin of feeling defeated the minute we take the last bite, it's not worth it.

Every time we face this moment we have to "consider it." We have to consider it because we will not feel joyful in the moment. We may feel deprived, jealous, and deserving. Or we may feel in the moment that the splurge will not affect us at all. But we have to consider it. Our feelings may be a true indicator of what we are facing, but they don't need to dictate our decisions.

We have to consider it and park our minds on the truth that our triumph in this trial matters. Triumph in this choice will produce a blessing. According to James, the blessing we have to consider is this: "that you may be mature and complete, not lacking anything" (James 1:4).

Oh sister, isn't this the heart of what we seek in our lives? I want to be mature and complete, not lacking anything. Therefore, I will persevere in the midst of this decision. I will choose the better option. And instead of feeling deprived when my salad arrives, I will rejoice. Because tucked in with the lettuce and grilled chicken is the realization I am capable of self-control. How good it is to consider the joy! And usually, by the time I'm leaving the restaurant having feasted on the healthier option, I also *feel* the joy.

Dear Lord, please help me when I feel tempted today. Triumph in this trial matters to me, and I desire to persevere with Your guidance. Help me to consider the joy and choose the better option. In Jesus' name. Amen.

Blessings Ahead

You know that the testing of your faith
produces perseverance.
Let perseverance finish its work.
(JAMES 1:3 – 4A)

Thought for the Day: Between any trial and the blessing that comes from that trial, there is a pathway I must walk — that pathway is perseverance.

Sandwiched between "consider it" and the blessing of becoming mature and complete that we read about last time in James is a key truth that can enable us to find joy in any circumstance:

> Consider it pure joy, my brothers and sisters, whenever you face trials of many kinds, because *you know that the testing of your faith produces perseverance. Let perseverance finish its work* so that you may be mature and complete, not lacking anything. (James 1:2 – 4, emphasis added)

Between any trial and the blessing that comes from that trial, there is a pathway we must walk — that pathway is perseverance.

Perseverance means having an urgency, firmness, resolve, and consistency. And, while the joy of the blessing may seem a long way off, signposts or mile markers of joy line the way. These will help us persevere with resolve and consistency if we "consider" them.

The first signpost we can consider in any circumstance, whether food related or otherwise, goes like this: "I might not be able to see the blessing right now, but this trial may be a *protection*—shielding me from something in the future that I may not see."

Let's consider what that protection might be. For example, I've realized that, had I never had a weight issue, I would have never been concerned about my health. In my mind, skinny equaled healthy. If I could have stayed skinny while living on a diet of chips and soda, I would have. I would never have acknowledged my body's needs for vitamins, fiber, healthy fats, and protein to regenerate healthy cells.

If my weight hadn't become an external indication of an internal situation, I never would have pursued healthy choices until I was facing a health crisis. Yes, this learning has helped me lose weight but, more importantly, it has forced me to learn about healthy eating as well as how to prevent disease, be more active, raise healthy children, and maybe even live longer. This gives me a measure of joy to persevere.

The second signpost we can consider to help us persevere is *provision*. Maybe God is providing me with many things I never expected to come from a trial. I've found camaraderie with my accountability friend that actually makes this food journey fun. I have found a surprising love of strawberries, hummus, snap peas, and many other good food choices. I can honestly say I've enjoyed discovering these wonderfully healthy foods at which I once turned up my nose. I crave what I eat. The more I provide my body with healthy foods, the more I crave healthy foods.

The final signpost we can consider along a path of perseverance is *process*. I have finally realized making lasting changes is a process. There are no quick fixes. There will be good days and bad days. But, most importantly, I've realized this isn't as much about losing the weight as it is gaining truth — the truth of who I am in Christ and how I am made for more than this constant, self-defeating struggle. It's the truth that reminds me a scale can measure my physical body but never my worth as a woman. And it's the truth that God loves me the way I am, but He loves me too much to leave me stuck in a place of defeat.

Through it all I've found a closeness to God I couldn't have imagined would have come out of a struggle with food. And, on top of everything else, God has used this trial to connect me with others and to help them with their weight struggles.

As we stop to consider the protection, the provision, and the process this trial has brought to us, we will find a measure of joy to persevere. Persevere — onward and upward, dear friend.

Dear Lord, even though I don't always understand Your ways, I can find joy in Your protection, Your provision, and Your process. I depend on Your strength to help me today. In Jesus' name. Amen.

Day 6

It's All in the Family

The Spirit himself testifies with our spirit
that we are God's children.

(ROMANS 8:16)

Thought for the Day: We are only one good choice away from being back on the path of perseverance. But no matter how far off the path or how long we have been on it, God is patient with us and loves us as a dearly beloved child—part of His family.

American humorist Erma Bombeck once said, "I come from a family where gravy is considered a beverage." Coming from the South, I can identify. Southern food culture taught me this: "If I love you, I will feed you—a lot!" And where did I often pile the most "love" on my plate? The church's covered-dish luncheons in the fellowship hall! Nowhere else could I get fried chicken, chicken-fried steak with sawmill gravy, sour cream mashed potatoes, with a side of spaghetti and meatballs. Then, of course, a "taste" of three different pies and some sweet tea to wash it all down. Boy, did it make the cooks happy to see my plate piled high! We called it "sharing the love."

So began my perception that food equals love. But like any unfaithful lover, food cannot love back. Overeating made me feel defeated and incapable. *Made to Crave* chronicles my one-sided love affair with food and the distress it caused me. That is, until my ever-expanding waistline and dismay caused me to direct my heart elsewhere.

As I began searching the Scriptures, I discovered how God can point our hearts to him: "May the Lord direct your hearts into God's love and Christ's perseverance" (2 Thessalonians 3:5). And I found some beautiful truths that help me to redirect my heart every day:

- *God's love never fails* (1 Corinthians 13:8). Even if we feel that we are weak and failing, God's love for us will never cease.

- *Nothing can separate us from God's love* (Romans 8:39). Not twenty, fifty, one-hundred, two-hundred pounds, or more — nothing will separate you from God's love.

- *Love is patient* (1 Corinthians 13:4). No matter how long we struggle to find victory in any area of our life, God is patient with us — continually providing His love, His comfort, His truth, and His power.

- *God's love is not based on our performance* (Romans 5:8). We may fall off the path of perseverance, but God's love has never been dependent on our actions, proven by the fact that He sent His son "while we were still sinners."

Yes, we are only one good choice away from being back on the path of perseverance. But no matter how far off the path or how long we are on it, God is patient with us and loves us as a dearly beloved child — part of His family (Romans 8:16 – 17; Galatians 4:7).

This reminds me of a touching story shared by my friend Karen Ehman, who lost over a hundred pounds in the first stage of her journey toward health. Her friend, Tammy, saw a "before" picture and was encouraging Karen enthusiastically when Karen's young son, Spencer, walked in. Tammy said, "Wow, Spencer, can you believe that was your mom? She's lost so much weight. Doesn't she look great?" In confusion, he looked back and forth between the photo and Karen and said, "Hmmm, they both look like Mama to me!"*

We are loved as God's special girls! No matter where you are in your struggle with healthy eating, God looks at you and says, "She still looks like my precious daughter to me!" He loves you just the way you are. But God loves you too much to leave you stuck in a state of defeat. You were made for so much more. You were made for victory.

Dear Lord, I am so thankful to be a part of Your family.
I know You love me no matter what. Please lead me today.
In Jesus' name. Amen.

---

*For more encouragement from my friend Karen Ehman, visit her at www.KarenEhman.com where she blogs daily.

Triggers

*I pray that you ... grasp how wide and long and high
and deep is the love of Christ ... that you may be filled
to the measure of all the fullness of God.*

(EPHESIANS 3:17–19)

Thought for the Day: The only way to negate an emotional eating
trigger is to match it with truth.

I was elated one day when the number on my scale finally dipped
below the plateau weight I'd been stuck at for two weeks. I did
a little happy dance and thought, "Finally, I'm making some real
progress in this journey. It's going to be such a great day. I'm super
motivated. Bring on the raw veggies. Nothing's gonna stop me
now!"

Too bad things didn't stay that way. Life, like math, can be
unpredictable.

I'm no math whiz, but I do remember there being these things
called polynomials. Polynomials are algebraic expressions that
include real numbers and variables. That's the way my food issues

are—they contain real numbers and variables. I suspect yours do as well. And while we must pay attention to the real numbers by eating less and moving more, we would do well to consider the variables in our lives as well.

Variables are those daily triggers we didn't account for but will detour even the best of intentions. Triggers can be as large as the stab of loneliness from a broken relationship or the memory of a childhood trauma. Triggers can be as small as a discipline "chat" with a teen out past curfew or stumbling across fresh doughnuts in the office break room. Any trigger can prompt the thought, "Life will be better if I eat that."

My blog readers have shared some of their triggers and the emotions behind them ...

- A "crazy day of carpool" or a "stressful project at work" brings subtle thoughts of "I've earned the right to this treat."
- "My mom hints that my house is messy," or "My husband works late and misses dinner—again," leads to "I give up on keeping myself all together, so why not give up on this food struggle too?"
- "There's birthday cake in the break room," or "My friends are all going out after work," leads us to believe that "It's not fair that everyone else can eat what they want and I can't."
- "I don't pay attention to what I eat when I'm bored or watching TV," or "I'm frustrated with my job," tells us that life feels unfulfilling, but "Life will be better if I eat this now!"

Notice, these triggers have nothing to do with physical hunger or the need for legitimate nourishment. They are lies that we've thought so routinely they've become well-worn paths to careless eating. Life is not made better because we overindulge in an unhealthy choice.

The best thing we can do in these triggered moments is to pause. Pause and ask ourselves, "Do I want to eat this right now because I need nourishment or because I'm feeling empty emotionally or spiritually?"

If I need nourishment, I can choose a healthy option. If I'm just feeling empty, I must realize food can fill my stomach but never my soul.

The only way to negate an emotional eating trigger is to match it with truth. The truth is this: "I'm not physically hungry right now, but I need to be filled in another way." The Bible tells us that we can be rooted in love, not emptiness; that we have power to choose truth; and that as we comprehend the love of Christ, we will be filled to the measure of all the fullness — not of that brownie — but of God (Ephesians 3:17 – 19). And here's the great thing about truth: it contains no variables! Truth is stable, secure, and a surefire way to get me through the unpredictable moments of life.

Take time to pause and use God's truths to challenge your triggers. And, when you're truly physically hungry, that pause will give you the moment you need to choose a healthy snack. Then you will be truly full!

Dear Lord, please help me to battle each of my triggers today with truth. Your truth. Moment by moment. I understand that food can fill my stomach but never my soul. Only You can fill my soul and I am thankful for that. In Jesus' name. Amen.

Isn't This Just a Small Thing?

Let the peace of Christ rule in your hearts,
since as members of one body you were called to peace.
And be thankful.

(COLOSSIANS 3:15)

Thought for the Day: My weight loss goal isn't a number on the scale. My real weight loss goal is peace.

Sometimes we Christian women think this food issue is a small thing. After all, gluttony seems to be overlooked as an acceptable Christian sin. It's not as big a deal to God as attitudes of selfishness, worldliness, or pride — or is it?

I considered my food struggle as a small thing in light of the bigger challenges of life. I can remember saying, "God, you can mess with my pride, you can mess with my anger, you can mess with my money, you can mess with my selfishness, you can mess with my frustration with my children, you can mess with the times I disrespect my husband ... you can mess with all that, but don't mess with my overeating." However, small things can easily become big things. Consider this example.

On January 15, 2009, Flight 1549 took off from New York's LaGuardia Airport with 155 occupants on board. The takeoff went fine, but three minutes later, at only three thousand feet, the plane encountered a flock of geese. Both engines shut down. Captain "Sully" Sullenberger had to make an immediate decision with life-or-death consequences. He made a miraculously successful emergency landing on the Hudson River. Those geese were small, but they brought down an entire plane. Small things can easily become big things.

I would do well to remember this principle.

Let's begin to acknowledge the "big" emotions that often accompany our "little" food struggle. I realized that I constantly bounced between feeling deprived and guilty; deprived, then guilty. My disgust and frustration with myself stripped me of the peace and joy that I wanted to be the hallmark of my life. Having peace *is* a big deal. Scripture tells us to let the peace of God rule in our hearts (Colossians 3:15). Isn't peace what we want in every area of our life — even our health?

Is your heart dominated by feelings of inadequacy, self-loathing, or defeat about your food struggles? Those are big emotions. Whenever we feel defeated by an issue, it can prevent us from following God completely. That's why my weight loss goal isn't a number on the scale. My real weight loss goal is peace. I knew I would be successful one day when I stood on the scale and I felt peace, no matter what the number said.

As we move through our healthy eating journey, the goal shouldn't just be a smaller waistline measurement, but a larger measure of peace. The apostle Paul puts it this way: "Let us therefore make every effort to do what leads to peace and to mutual edification. Do not destroy the work of God for the sake of food"

(Romans 14:19 – 20a). In other words, don't let a small thing become a big thing.

I often ask myself this pivotal question before making a food choice: *Will this choice add to my peace or steal from it?* Remember, nothing tastes as good as peace feels.

Dear Lord, Your peace is what I plead for today. I don't want my focus to be on food, a number on the scale, insecurity, or inadequacy. I want my focus to be on You. That is where I will find true peace. In Jesus' name. Amen.

Day 9

Compromise vs. Promise

"The thief comes only to steal and kill and destroy;
I have come that [you] may have life, and have it to the full."
(JOHN 10:10)

Thought for the Day: What happens when you take the "com" off of compromise? You are left with a promise. A promise you are meant to live.

I headed straight to the pantry. No doubt about it, this was an occasion when comfort food was completely justifiable.

My son had come to me scared and admitted that he had compromised his standards and gone too far with his girlfriend. They hadn't crossed every line, but enough that he knew they were headed in a dangerous direction. He wanted help processing what to do. We considered this definition:

> com•pro•mise (kom´prə•mīz´)
>
> 1. to expose or make vulnerable
> 2. to make an unfavorable concession or indulgence
> 3. to weaken

This is exactly the way he felt—that they had exposed their relationship to emotions they were not ready to handle. They had indulged in an area God wanted to preserve, yet the world told them they deserved. And, it had weakened their relationship.

We sat on the back deck and processed the situation together. I said, "What happens when you delete 'com' from the word *compromise*? You're left with a 'promise.'" I shared that he was made for more than compromise. He was made for God's promises in every area of his life.

We read many of the empowering Scripture verses I've included in this book, seeking to filter every part of this situation through God's truth. In the end, he and his girlfriend came to the realization they needed to break up. It's really hard to put things in reverse after certain lines have been crossed.

I walked back into the house after that conversation with two things running through my brain. I was thrilled my son came to me to talk about such a sensitive issue. What an honor to breathe truth into his physical struggle.

But I also felt a little panicked at the realities of parenting an older teenager. And this feeling convinced me I had to have some comfort food! As I loaded my arms full of treats, I turned and saw my son standing on the other side of the kitchen. I was suddenly struck by a gut-wrenching question. How could I expect my son to apply truth to the area of his greatest physical struggle, but refuse to apply it to my area of greatest physical struggle?

This question struck deep. If I wanted to model what it looks like to live out truth in my physical struggles, I would have to break up with unhealthy choices. I admit that indulging in chips and brownies is a small concession compared to a young couple compromising their purity. But if one indulgence leads to two, and that leads to other indulgences, then the downward spiral is quite similar.

And whether we are talking about having premarital sex or other compromises that make us feel defeated, we must remember a crucial truth. We were made for God's promises that lead to an abundant life of truth, strength, and joy. Satan's purpose is to compromise God's promised best: "The thief's purpose is to steal and kill and destroy. My purpose is to give [you] a rich and satisfying life" (John 10:10 NLT). Don't allow this thief to weaken, expose, or make you vulnerable. Don't compromise. Refuse to accept less than the peace and abundant life God has promised you.

Listen for this lie the thief will often whisper: "This will make you feel wonderful!" Combat this lie with this: "You are a liar and a destroyer, Satan. Yes, this may feel wonderful in the moment, but how will I feel in the morning? I will not let your poisonous invitation for pleasure in the moment derail and defeat me. I am not made for compromise. I am made to live the reality of God's promises."

This is true for my son. This is true for me. This is true for you, dear friend.

Dear Lord, I know You will lead me to an abundant life of truth, strength, and joy. Protect me from the enemy's derailing distractions today. Help me to live out Your promises instead. In Jesus' name. Amen.

Why Do We Crave?

Do not love the world or anything in the world. . . .
For everything in the world — the lust of the flesh,
the lust of the eyes, and the pride of life —
comes not from the Father but from the world.

(1 JOHN 2:15 – 16)

Thought for the Day: While Eve focused on the object of her temptation, Jesus kept his focus on God's truth. What matters most to me?

Think about the definition of the word *craving*. How would you define it? Dictionary.com defines craving as something you long for, want greatly, desire eagerly, and beg for. God made us to crave so we'd always desire more of Him.

Don't read over that last sentence too quickly. God made us to crave — to desire eagerly, want greatly, and long for Him. But Satan wants to do everything possible to replace our craving for God with something else. I like how the New Living Translation puts this:

Do not love this world nor the things it offers you, . . . for the world offers only a craving for physical pleasure, a craving for everything we see, and pride in our achievements and possessions. These are not from the Father, but are from this world. (1 John 2:15–16 NLT)

The cravings of the world are misplaced physical desires—such as issues with food or for sex outside of marriage. In other words, trying to meet our physical needs outside the will of God. A craving for everything we see means being enamored by material things. And lastly, pride in achievements and possessions describes someone chasing what brings feelings of significance.

This passage details three ways Satan tries to lure us away from loving God. And Satan used these very same tactics the first time he tempted humankind through Eve:

When the woman saw that the fruit of the tree was good for food [physical craving] and pleasing to the eye [material craving], and also desirable for gaining wisdom [significance craving], she took some and ate it. (Genesis 3:6)

Eve kept her focus on the object of her desire. The Scriptures give us no indication she tried to check in with God or Adam. She didn't walk away and truly consider this choice. And she certainly didn't take time to consider the consequences.

She saw it. She wanted it. She bought the lie. She took it. And she suffered for it.

Interestingly, Satan later applied the same three tactics he used with Eve when he tempted Jesus (Matthew 4).

Physical craving: Satan appealed to Jesus' physical need for food (Matthew 4:3). Jesus had been fasting, so of course He was hungry. It's comforting for me to know Jesus felt the pangs of hunger yet resisted because He was fasting. He didn't want to get His physical needs met outside the will of God.

Material craving: The devil promised Jesus all the kingdoms He could see if He would bow down to the god of materialism (Matthew 4:8–9). It's hard to resist the splendor of the world. But Jesus was enamored with God's eternity, not the world's temporary imitations. He didn't want to get His material needs met outside the will of God.

Significance craving: The enemy enticed Jesus to prove His significance by forcing God to command angels to save Him (Matthew 4:5–6). The lure of doing something that will make one look good, feel powerful, and be elevated in the eyes of others is so enticing. But Jesus' security came from His identity as a child of God, not His human achievements. He didn't want to get His emotional significance needs met outside the will of God.

While Eve focused on the object of her temptation, Jesus kept His focus on God's truth. He refuted each of Satan's lures with Scripture.

He saw it. He wanted God more. He quoted truth. He resisted. And He was rewarded for it.

When we face our own cravings, will we be like Eve, focusing on our object of desire? Or will we be like Jesus, pausing, reciting truth, and remembering what matters most? Temporary satisfaction or unending contentment? Giving in to the cravings of this world or following the love and the will of God? Two powerful examples. Two vastly different outcomes.

Dear Lord, please help me as I struggle with physical, material, and significance cravings. I know that only You can bring me lasting contentment for my cravings. Help me to pause today and reflect on what matters most. In Jesus' name. Amen.

A Grace Place

Let us then approach God's throne of grace with confidence,
so that we may receive mercy
and find grace to help us in our time of need.
(HEBREWS 4:16)

Thought for the Day:
God is asking me to go to a new place — a place of grace!

I once wondered if God ever got tired of my issues — those recurring failings and sins I couldn't ever seem to conquer. Throughout my lifelong struggle with emotional eating, I whined to God, got mad at God, and often ignored God. And I worried I was going to use up all my grace with God. I felt He would be justified to say, "Enough! Go away. I'm tired of your issues. Figure it out for yourself!"

That is, until I read again the "first story" of God's grace with fresh eyes. We often think of God's grace beginning at the cross. But as I read through the Scripture from the point of view of someone struggling with food issues, I saw a revelation of God's grace right from the start in Genesis.

Adam and Eve disobeyed God by eating from the forbidden tree and ushered sin in to the world. God handed down the consequences of their actions, which included banishment from the Garden of Eden (Genesis 3).

It must have seemed to them that they had pushed past the boundaries of God's grace. After all, He was sending them out of the garden. Whenever I've read that story, I thought they had to leave paradise because God was punishing them. God was disappointed in them. God was giving them what they deserved.

But I was wrong. Their relocation was not a place of abandonment — it was a place of grace.

You see, there were two special trees in the Garden of Eden. One was the tree of the knowledge of good and evil; this was the one with the forbidden fruit. The other was the tree of life. This was the one that gave Adam and Eve perpetual life — no diseases, no death, no sagging body parts. (Okay I'm not sure about that last benefit, but I'm banking on this reality in heaven.)

Anyhow.

When they ate of the tree of the knowledge of good and evil, sin entered in. Sin corrupted everything. And at that point, it was God's absolute love and most tender mercy that ushered Adam and Eve out of the garden. Not His anger or retaliation.

They had to leave. If they'd been allowed to stay, they would have kept eating from the tree of life and lived forever, wallowing in sin. Wallowing in all the brokenness sin brings with it: disease, fear, heartbreak, separation from God. An unending life of shame and sin would have been their fate. And God couldn't stand that for the people He loved.

So, His love made them leave and allowed them to die. So that they could experience the resurrected life His Son would one day provide. Brokenness to redemption.

God did not run out of grace at the dawn of humankind. And He will not run out of grace for you or for me. He does not want us to ever stay in a perpetual state of sin and despair. We were not created with a food struggle or physical cravings because God is angry at us. It is because He loves us so much that He allows our struggle with food to be a physical indication of a spiritual situation. God is asking for us to go to a new place as well—and it is a place of grace!

Receive grace and let it wash away all shame and guilt from every unhealthy choice you've ever regretted and fretted over. Yes, there is work to do and progress to be made, but we will walk from here with a clean slate.

This grace and the unfathomable depth of God's love settle me. Breathes hope into my dread. And trust into my doubts. So when I stumble along on this journey, I know this grace is there for me, and I will come running back. And once again, it will give me a soft place to land.

Dear Lord, thank You for Your grace. Thank You for Your love. Thank You for never giving up on me. Help me to live as Your grateful daughter today. In Jesus' name. Amen.

Emotional Emptiness

Taste and see that the LORD is good;
blessed is the one who takes refuge in him.
(PSALM 34:8)

Thought for the Day: Somewhere behind all of the numbers, a less measurable force is at work within me. It takes the form of emptiness or lack.

Sometimes people struggle with food because they eat too much of the wrong kinds of foods, and they consume more calories than their bodies need. The physics of dieting are pretty straightforward.

While this is as true for me as for the next person, some things make the prospect of losing weight a little more complicated for me. Somewhere behind all of the numbers, a less measurable force is at work within me. It's emptiness or lack.

As I trace my fingers back across the timeline of my life, I remember times when spiritual and emotional emptiness left me vulnerable. This emotional emptiness stemmed from coming home from school one day and being told, "Your daddy's gone."

Many life struggles since then have left me feeling vulnerable and empty as well.

Emptiness demands to be filled. And when I couldn't figure out how to fill what my heart was lacking, my stomach was more than willing to offer a few suggestions. Food became a comfort I could turn on and off like a faucet. It was easy. It was filling. It was available. It became a pattern. And somehow, each time my heart felt a little empty, my stomach picked up on the cues and suggested I feed it instead.

Many times my overstuffed stomach could be traced back to an empty place in my heart, and that, in turn, could be traced back to my thought life. It's so easy to park our minds in bad spots. To dwell and rehash and wish things were different. But to think on hard things keeps us in hard spots and only serves to deepen feelings of emotional emptiness. This is where pity parties are held, and we all know pity parties demand an abundance of high-calorie delights, eaten and eaten some more. But pity parties are a cruel way to entertain, for they leave behind a deeper emptiness than that with which we started.

At some point, I came to realize overeating was adding to my hurt, not soothing it. We have the choice to either let those past hurts continue to haunt and damage us or to allow forgiveness to pave the way for the new life and lasting changes we desire.

I can't go back and change the things that happened to me in the past. But I can forgive. I can refuse to let my abusers and accusers hurt me more by sending me on emotional eating binges. So, one by one, I've gone to those memories and said, "Yes, this is a circumstance of my life, but it doesn't define who I am."

And I can forgive myself with the same statement. Satan says,

"Your past mistakes are horrible!" And I reply, "Yes, these mistakes are things I wish I could change, but they don't define who I am."

Rather than dwelling on wounds that leave us feeling emotionally empty, we can learn to look for whatever is true, noble, right, pure, lovely, admirable, excellent, and praiseworthy in life (Philippians 4:8). When I park my mind and heart on thoughts that *refresh* me instead of ones that *depress* me, I am filled. Like the psalmist reminds us, "Taste and see that the LORD is good" (Psalm 34:8).

Dear Lord, help me claim these truths as my own, help me to look for what is right and pure. I am going to look at my situations and understand that they are circumstances of my life, but they don't define me. Only You define me. And You love me, Lord. I proclaim this truth today. In Jesus' name. Amen.

Honestly

Be diligent in these matters;
give yourself wholly to them,
so that everyone may see your progress.
(1 TIMOTHY 4:15)

Thought for the Day: It is possible to rise up, do battle with our issues, and, using the Lord's strength in us, defeat them — spiritually, physically, and mentally — to the glory of God.

I think we all get to a place sometimes where we have to honestly assess, "How am I doing?"

It's not really a conversation I have with a friend or family member. It's one of those middle-of-the-night contemplations where there's no one to fool. There's no glossing over the realities staring me in the face.

I know certain things about myself need to change, but it's easier to make excuses than tackle them head on. Rationalizations are so appealing:

I'm good in every other area.

I make so many sacrifices already.

I need comfort in this season of life — I'll deal with it later.

I just can't give this up.

The Bible doesn't specifically say this is wrong.

It's not really a problem; if I wanted to make a change, I could — I just don't want to right now.

Oh for heaven's sake, everyone has issues; so what if this is mine?

And on and on and on.

Excuses always get me nowhere fast. That's why a few years ago I had to get honest in the area of healthy eating. Even if that's not your issue, I suspect these same scripts of rationalization have played out in your mind over other things.

So, the cycle continues day after day, week after week, year after year.

One day, I finally decided I didn't want to spend a lifetime in this cycle.

Nothing changed until I made the choice to change. I had to want it — spiritually, physically, and mentally. The battle really is in all three areas.

Spiritually: The Bible tells us to set our minds and our hearts on things above (Colossians 3:1–5). To do this, I have to put to death whatever belongs to my earthly nature, which is anything that sets itself up as an idol in my life. Idolatry is trying to get my needs met outside the will of God.

I couldn't deny it. This described food for me at times. More often than I cared to admit, I turned to food when I should have turned to God.

Physically: I couldn't keep my weight stable in a medically healthy range for any period of time. I would lose weight, but then I would always gain it back. And then to top it all off, when a doctor did some tests to determine my body mass index (BMI), my body fat percentage had crept up to the "danger" category.

What?! I knew I was feeling sluggish and frustrated by the extra weight, but no one would have looked at me and thought I was at risk. Except now a doctor was telling me that if I didn't make some changes, I could be in trouble.

I needed a healthy eating plan, not a fad diet. I needed a plan that would help me make realistic changes to improve my overall health and help me shed the excess weight the right way.

Mentally: Don't settle. Don't compromise. Remember what we discussed in Day 9 about cutting the "com" off of the word *compromise*? You're left with a "promise." We were made for more than compromise. We were made for God's promises in all areas of life. I am made for more than a vicious cycle of eating, gaining, stressing; eating, gaining, stressing ...

For the sake of my emotional health, it was time to be honest with myself.

Remember, as a Jesus girl, it is possible to rise up, do battle with our issues, and, using the Lord's strength in us, defeat them — spiritually, physically, and mentally — to the glory of God.

Dear Lord, help me to be courageous enough to speak honestly to You and to myself about areas where I'm giving in to compromise. Show me how to rely on Your strength for more self-discipline in my life — not for my glory, but for Yours. In Jesus' name. Amen.

Finish the Work

I tell you, open your eyes and look at the fields!
They are ripe for harvest.

(JOHN 4:35B)

Thought for the Day:
Food can fill my stomach but never my soul.

If you've attended many Christian women's events, you've probably heard the story of the Samaritan woman told from just about every possible angle. If I hear someone start to speak about her at a conference, I'll admit my brain begs me to tune out and daydream about tropical places or items I need to add to my grocery list.

It's not that I don't like her story. I do. It's just that I've heard it so many times I find myself doubting there could possibly be anything fresh left to say about it. But in all my years of hearing about the Samaritan woman, reading her story, and feeling like I know it, I missed something. Something really big.

Right smack dab in the middle of one of the longest recorded interactions Jesus has with a woman, He starts talking about food.

Food! And I'd never picked up on it before. I somehow missed Jesus' crucial teaching that our bodies must have two kinds of nourishment: physical and spiritual.

Just as I must have physical food for my body to survive, I have to have spiritual food for my soul to thrive. Jesus says, "My food ... is to do the will of him who sent me and to finish his work" (John 4:34). And then He goes on to say, "I tell you, open your eyes and look at the fields! They are ripe for harvest" (John 4:35b).

There is a bigger plan here! Don't get distracted by physical food. Don't think physical food can satisfy the longing of your soul. Only Jesus can do this. Our souls were created to crave Him and love others to Him. So many people are waiting to hear the message of your calling. Don't get stuck in defeat and held back from it.

In the midst of offering salvation to the Samaritan woman, Jesus seems to wander off on this tangent about food. But it's not a tangent at all. Actually, it fits perfectly. It relates directly to the core issue of spiritual malnutrition. Specifically, it's about trying to use food to fill not only the physical void of our stomachs but also the spiritual void of our souls. For years, I've been physically overweight but spiritually underweight. How crucial it is for us to remember:

> Food can fill our stomachs but never our souls.
>
> Possessions can fill our houses but never our hearts.
>
> Sex can fill our nights but never our hunger for love.
>
> Children can fill our days but never our identities.

Jesus wants us to know only He can fill us and truly satisfy us. He really wants us to really believe that.

Only by being filled with authentic soul food from Jesus — following Him and telling others about Him — will our souls ever be truly satisfied. And breaking free from consuming thoughts about food allows us to see and pursue our calling with more confidence and clarity.

Dear Lord, I know that it is true that only You can fill me.
I acknowledge that You are the Lord of my life. I want
to please You today in all that I do. Help me to follow You.
In Jesus' name. Amen.

Day
15

Unsolicited Feedback

*Since, then, you have been raised with Christ, set your hearts on
things above, where Christ is, seated at the right hand of God.
Set your minds on things above, not on earthly things.*

(COLOSSIANS 3:1–2)

Thought for the Day: Don't let people's compliments go to your
head, and don't let their criticisms go to your heart. The degree to
which you do either of these things is the degree to which you'll be
ruled by what other people think of you.

Anytime we put ourselves "out there" in any way, we can feel
exposed—whether it's going on a job interview, presenting a holi-
day meal, or waiting for guests to RSVP to our party. I felt deeply
exposed when I finally said out loud to someone else, "I'm starting
a new healthy eating plan."

I was concerned that others might roll their eyes and think,
"There she goes dieting again." I anticipated the eerie feeling that
friends and skeptics would now pass judgment on my every bite.

Even well-meaning encouragement or questions can be embar-
rassing when it calls attention to an area of struggle. A friend once

asked in front of a group if she could have my size 16 slacks, now that I was wearing a smaller size. While she meant to highlight my successful weight loss, a different response ran through my mind: "Now everyone knows the number I previously thought I'd hidden behind fashionable pleats and tunic sweaters!" In addition, the brief suspicion struck me that everyone was really wondering if I would gain all the weight back again. Some people call this insecurity. I call it normal. So, what's a girl to do?

Don't let people's compliments go to your head, and don't let their criticisms go to your heart. The degree to which you do either of these things is the degree to which you'll be ruled by what other people think of you. And, boy, I know from experience how dangerous it is to build the stability of my identity on the fickle opinions of others.

Each day, let God whisper into your heart the truth of who you are—and whose you are. Filter the opinions of others through the reality that just because they think it doesn't make it true. Be brave enough to accept *negative* feedback as a possible call to action, but not a definition of your identity. And while you enjoy the *positive* feedback, refuse to get bloated by it.

We must rise above the chatter of the world, place our identities in the un-shifting grace of God, and keep our hearts tuned to the reassuring whispers of Jesus.

Dear Lord, I struggle caring too much about the opinions of others. I beg You to please whisper words of truth into my heart and mind today. Protect me from both the bad and good opinions of others as I am reminded that only Your opinion counts. In Jesus' name. Amen.

And I Thought
There Was No Good

And we know that in all things
God works for the good of those who love him,
who have been called according to his purpose.
(ROMANS 8:28)

Thought for the Day: Whether your issues are the same as mine or not, all of us Jesus girls have struggles of some kind. We all fall short in some manner.

If you would have told me ten years ago that God could bring good out of my weight issues and food struggles, I would have seriously doubted you. And then, when you weren't looking, I would have rolled my eyes. A soul rubbed raw from years of trying and failing does not want to hear, "Eventually, good will come from this."

What I wanted was something to magically fix my issues. I wanted to be naturally thin like my sister. I wanted to feel "not fat." I would have cared less about some elusive, eventual good. My jeans didn't fit. Even my sweatpants didn't fit. I felt horrible.

I couldn't stay committed to a healthy eating plan to save my life. And I saw no evidence of hope on the horizon.

Maybe you've been there with your food issues and weight struggles. Maybe you're there right now. May I be a ray of hope to you today? Whether your issues are the same as mine or not, all of us Jesus girls have struggles of some kind. We all fall short in some manner. And we all need to know more about this "good" mentioned in Romans 8:28.

Not long ago I received a letter that confirmed this truth. The writer's honest confession was like heaven's salve, soothing my soul and spreading "this working of good." Somehow God took my simple words in *Made to Crave*, scrawled from deep places I thought were no good, and brought this good from it:

> I just want to say thank you. I've had a severe eating disorder since 1978. I became a Christian in 2002, but never could fully surrender my eating disorder to the Lord. Through your book, the Holy Spirit is empowering me as I never thought possible. I've had seven days of no binging or purging. This may not seem like a high number to you, but after thirty-three years with this addiction, this is amazing. Praise God!

May this be a glimpse of hope in the midst of whatever struggle is trying to bring you down today. It is a picture of the reality that God's Word is true — always true. God does work for the good, in all things, every single thing — even our most raw and seemingly impossible things. But we must "know" it even when we don't feel it, and let God have His way.

And we know it, even if we don't feel it, that in all things — even the ones I can't fathom being used for good — God works for the good. *He* works for the good. My job is to walk with Him day by day. His job is to work the good.

Dear Lord, help me to look for the good in my situation today. I pray that as I look at my eating struggles, I will glimpse the good You are able to bring from it. I desire healing and hope for my road ahead. Please be with me. In Jesus' name. Amen.

The War against My Soul

Dear friends, I urge you,
as foreigners and exiles, to abstain from sinful desires,
which wage war against your soul.

(1 PETER 2:11)

Thought for the Day: Being ruled by anything other than God is something He takes quite seriously. And so should we.

For years, I refused to think of my struggle with healthy eating as anything more than just a physical issue. I didn't pray about it. I didn't apply biblical insights to it. And I certainly didn't ask God for help. I just wallowed in my lack of self-control.

This issue was too small for God, but too big for me.

When I began connecting my physical struggle with spiritual insight, I wasn't convinced that God really cared about my bulging body. Was I merely being vain to want to be thinner? Was I wasting my time on things of this world when I went to the gym? Was I just a foolish, Jesus-chasing girl who mistakenly believed my desires to please Him with this food battle would somehow help me grow closer to Him?

As I studied the Scriptures, I knew I had my answer from God: "Dear friends, I urge you, as foreigners and exiles, to abstain from sinful desires, which wage war against your soul" (1 Peter 2:11).

My ever-increasing weight and poor food choices were wreaking havoc on my body. But that wasn't all. My desperate struggle, hopelessness, and uncontrollable food cravings were waging war against my soul. These were some of the whispers being hissed in my ear: *You'll never be free from this battle. You will always bounce from feeling deprived when you're dieting to feeling guilty when you're splurging. Victory isn't possible!*

When Satan holds up food in front us and says these things, we must see that an inappropriate relationship with food can be the lure he uses to draw us away from God. Satan may also use alcohol, unedifying media, inappropriate friendships, overspending, or any other means to lead us into a place where we feel self-control isn't possible. He's not choosy about the method, just the result.

One day while reading Psalm 23, I listed all the things the Lord does for me:

- He leads me.
- He restores me.
- He guides me.
- He is with me.
- He comforts me.
- He fills me.
- He satisfies me.

As I read back over my list, a series of questions shocked me: Do I rely on the Lord in these ways or do I rely on food in these ways? Do I honestly turn to God or turn to food? Do I seek to be comforted, filled, and satisfied in the depths of my soul with God, or food? My answers made me cry.

Being ruled by anything other than God is something He takes quite seriously. And so should we. For years, I was overweight physically but underweight spiritually. Tying those two things together has finally allowed me to see why so many other diets failed. I needed to dig past the surface to the real heart and soul of my issues.

In the process of that soul digging, I realized how amazing it is to serve a compassionate God—a God who knew food would be a major stumbling block, keeping many of His children from wholeheartedly pursuing Him. So He's given us great gifts in the Holy Spirit, Jesus, and the Bible to help us.

Start and finish your day with Bible reading. Pray before you eat —even snacks. Listen to that spiritual gut check when you're about to eat something. Choose the healthy option. Stop before you're overly full. Eat slowly. Refuse to stuff and gorge. Stay on a slower eating pace while enjoying conversation with others.

Yes, I want to get healthy. Yes, I want to lose weight. But this journey is about so much more. In the end, pursuing health helps my heart to feel closer to Jesus and more ready to receive what He wants for me each day.

Dear Lord, it is true. My food struggles at times wage a war against my soul. Because of this one overwhelming struggle, I often feel defeated in other areas of my life as well. As I seek You today, please give me the strength I need. Thank You. In Jesus' name. Amen.

Well Pleased

And a voice from heaven said,
"This is my Son, whom I love;
with him I am well pleased."
(MATTHEW 3:17)

Thought for the Day: Daily, hourly, and moment by moment, I must stand in the reality of my God-given identity.

When I was a young child, before my dad abandoned our family, I dressed in my best dress and twirled before him. I was desperate to hear words of love and affirmation he never gave me. In my teen years, I tried to earn his attention by performing well and getting good grades. But no matter how well I performed, my dad didn't stay. He didn't love me. He didn't approve of me.

This kind of hurt sinks deep into the longing heart of a girl.

It's probably no surprise that I used the same approach with my heavenly Father. I thought I had to perform for His approval. For years, I did the religious dance of Bible study, ministry leadership, prayer, and service to gain God's approval. Instead of doing these things because I was loved, I did them *so that* I'd be loved. It's important to be mindful of this dynamic so we don't link our food struggles to a similar kind of performance mentality.

Have you ever struggled with feeling like a "good Christian" when you exercised self-control and feeling like a "bad Christian" when you didn't? We must chat about this. While we do want to gain spiritual perspectives while losing the weight, we must resist slipping into performance mode.

In the Gospels, God makes a powerful statement about Jesus: "This is my Son, whom I love; with him I am well pleased" (Matthew 3:17).

I found new perspective in this passage when I realized that Jesus had not yet gone to the cross, performed miracles, or led the masses. His Father affirmed Jesus' identity *before* Jesus started His public ministry. Jesus heard God, believed God, and remained filled.

In Christ, God has given us a new identity (Romans 6:4). But, unlike Christ, we tend to forget who we are and to fill our lives with endless activities to prove our worth and significance. We do this to earn love and approval from other people as well as from God. Our humanity makes us hungry people. It is similar to the phenomenon of being satisfied with a large dinner one evening only to wake up the next morning feeling famished. Truth comes in and fills us up, but we can't expect one serving of truth to feed us for a lifetime. Our emotional cracks, crevices, and life circumstances are like drain holes that leak the truth and leave behind only hollowness.

Therefore, we must stand moment by moment in the truth of our identity before we resume our daily activities and even our healthy eating efforts. Grasp the truth and rub it in deep. Let it fill the drain holes that leach away your significance. Hear God say,

"You are my daughter, whom I love; with you I am well pleased." Well pleased because of who you are, not what you do. Well pleased because of an unfathomable, unconditional love — a love not earned but simply given.

And isn't it interesting that right after we read God's affirmation of Jesus in Matthew 3, the very next chapter starts off with Jesus being tempted with food while fasting in the desert? But because Jesus was filled with truth, He didn't engage the enemy. Remember? He deflected Satan's lies by repeatedly quoting Scripture. He remained steady, believing who He was and whose He was. His identity was established before His ministry activities began.

When we know our identity *before* we jump into activity, we don't have to guess how to handle the vicious lies of the enemy. We don't need to displace God with inappropriate physical pleasure or material comforts. We don't need to crave the acceptance of others. Because in God we are loved, accepted, and whole.

Oh, may this statement straight from God be inscribed, engraved, and tattooed in the most permanent of ways on our hearts: "Well pleased ... well pleased ... well pleased."

God loves you, sweet sister. Rest in this reality today.

Dear Lord, I don't often feel that You are well pleased with me. Help me to change my perspective and remember that You love me regardless of what I do. You loved me before I was even born. And You are well pleased with me now. Help me to live like I believe this today. In Jesus' name. Amen.

Creating New Space
for Growth

Then [Jesus] said to them all:
"Whoever wants to be my disciple must deny themselves
and take up their cross daily and follow me."
(LUKE 9:23)

Thought for the Day: If I want to grow closer to God, I have to distance myself from whatever is distracting me.

Over the years, I have felt the desire to become more than just a checklist Christian. I've wrestled with the question, "How can I grow closer to God?" And I wasn't looking for the plastic Christian answers: Go to church. Read the Bible. Don't cuss. Be nice. Pray.

Those are all good things. Things we should do. But we can do all those things and still have hearts far from God. I want connection. I want communion. I want closeness.

The New Living Translation puts Jesus' words in Luke 9:23 like this: "If any of you wants to be my follower, you must turn from your selfish ways, take up your cross daily, and follow me." I want this kind of all-out pursuit with God. But what does this look like in today's culture?

I think part of what it means is breaking old habits to create space in my heart for new growth.

In reality, God desires our sacrifice— our turning from selfish ways—not for His benefit, but for ours. For instance, I stopped watching TV for a season. I realized I was turning on the TV when I felt most depleted—and when I'm most depleted, I soak up deeply whatever I take in. Why would I want to soak in deeply the entertainment of this world and not things that breathe life back into me? I broke the old habit of watching television and created space in my heart for new growth.

Another example is my commitment to do nothing else each morning—including checking my phone or turning on the computer —before I open up God's Word. I used to wake up eager to tune in to the world. I'd soon be sucked into answering this email, reading that Twitter post, and returning phone calls. Before I knew it, half my day was gone, and I hadn't let God prepare my heart for any of it. So I broke the old habit and created space in my heart for new growth.

Right now, I'm intentionally sacrificing sugar and processed foods that turn into sugar once consumed. Yes, I want to maintain my weight loss. But this journey is so much more than just that. It really is about learning to tell myself no and learning to make wiser choices daily. And somehow becoming a woman of self-discipline honors God and helps me live the godly characteristic of self-control. Giving up sugar was hard at first—really hard, like crying-big-crocodile-tears hard. But I broke the old habit and created space in my heart for growth.

Am I saying all my Jesus girlfriends need to do the same? No more TV? No checking your computer and phone first thing in the morning? No sugar? Nope. These aren't things I think everyone needs to do. They were personal practices for my own benefit. I'm not asking you to follow *me*; I'm saying to follow wholeheartedly after God. Ask Him. Seek Him. Do what He tells you.

If we want to grow closer to God, we'll have to distance ourselves from whatever is distracting us. Break the old habit and create space in your heart for new growth. And closeness will soon bloom.

Dear Lord, I realize that You do not need me. I need You. But I don't often live each day understanding this. Far too often, I forge ahead and battle my issues without You. I want to grow closer to You, to live each day with You. Help me to remember You will never leave me. Thank You for loving me. In Jesus' name. Amen.

Day
20

Worship

Therefore, I urge you, brothers and sisters,
in view of God's mercy,
to offer your bodies as a living sacrifice,
holy and pleasing to God—
this is your true and proper worship.
(ROMANS 12:1)

Thought for the Day:
What we fix our attention, heart, and mind on
is what we'll worship.

What we fix our attention, heart, and mind on is what we'll worship. What we worship becomes magnified. And what is magnified will consume us and perpetuate more and more worship.

If we think about this in light of food struggles, we can see how easily incessant thoughts of food can crowd out thoughts of God. We must beware: God made us to consume food, but food was never supposed to consume us. We were made to crave—focus on, magnify, and worship—God. God alone.

The author of Psalms beautifully illustrates why worshiping

God is what we were made to do: "Your ways, God, are holy. What god is as great as our God? You are the God who performs miracles; you display your power among the peoples" (Psalm 77:13–14).

The psalmist also describes how God performed miracles, such as dividing the sea, leading His people out of captivity, bringing water from a rock, and giving the Israelites everything they needed to survive (Psalm 78:12–16). But they eventually forgot all that God had done for them:

> But they continued to sin against him, rebelling in the wilderness against the Most High. *They willfully put God to the test by demanding the food they craved....* When the LORD heard [their complaints], he was furious. (Psalm 78:17–18, 21a, emphasis added)

"They willfully put God to the test by demanding the food they craved." Now this is a line I need to read over and over.

Honestly, many of the verses from Psalm 78 hit me hard, because they so specifically address inappropriate cravings and the reality of how God feels about them. And the truths in this chapter answer so many questions about why this journey has been such a crucial part of my spiritual growth. Like the Israelites, I have tasted God's provision and the deep satisfaction of His love. I too have seen God work in mighty ways. I've been led through the impossible. He's guided me through trials. He's brought living water to replace my dried-up places. He's given me everything, and I don't want to forget.

Not with my mind, not with my soul, not with my heart, and certainly not with my body.

So, how do we make the shift from worshiping food to worshiping God?

We stop *intending* to worship God and start getting *intentional*. One small act of obedience is better than a hundred good intentions. "Therefore, I urge you, brothers and sisters, in view of God's mercy, to offer your bodies as a living sacrifice, holy and pleasing to God—this is your true and proper worship" (Romans 12:1). The words, "I urge you," prompt me to know this isn't something I should "intend" to consider; offering my body to the Lord as an act of worship is something I need to get intentional about implementing.

What are some good choices you've been intending to make? How can you get intentional with those things today? This week? This month? This year? Think how good you'll feel to look back on this day as the day you started walking toward victory.

Indeed, what we fix our attention, heart, and mind on is what we'll worship. What we worship becomes magnified. And what is magnified will consume us and perpetuate more and more worship.

Dear Lord, please help me to identify my inappropriate cravings today. I offer them back to You and ask You to take them as my act of worship today. I want to crave You and only You. In Jesus' name. Amen.

But Victory Seems
So Far Away

*Rejoice always, pray continually,
give thanks in all circumstances;
for this is God's will for you in Christ Jesus.*

(1 THESSALONIANS 5:16–18)

Thought for the Day: I can't control my circumstances, but I can control my choices. Setting mini goals—physically and spiritually—positions me for victory.

There are days I don't feel victorious. Like the day when the upstairs toilet clogged and flooded my kitchen ceiling. Or the day I got stuck in traffic, yelled at my kids, and missed an important meeting. Those are the days when my long-term goals to get healthy don't feel as important as my need for immediate comfort. I just want to blow my healthy eating plan out of frustration with something gooey, sweet, and cream laden.

I bet you've had something occur this week that doesn't make you feel very victorious either. A sick child, a missed deadline, tension in a friendship, or a number on the scale that almost made you cry. I understand. But may I encourage you? Even in the midst of trying circumstances and bad days, you can be victorious.

You can be victorious even when the distance between your present reality and your desired goal seems so far apart.

How?

Set mini-goals. Losing twenty, fifty, one hundred pounds, or more can seem so far away. And faraway goals are hard to hang onto when life drains us and it feels like those French fries sure could fill us.

Set mini-goals physically by getting a strategy for making healthy choices. How can you prepare now to drink eight glasses of water today? What is a healthy snack option you'll turn to when those afternoon salty and sugary cravings start calling? Are you going out to eat at a restaurant? Use the Internet to look up the nutritional information for their menu so you can make informed healthy choices. If hit with an unexpected temptation today, what healthy go-to script or Bible verse can you arm yourself with in advance to combat justifications and compromises?

Each mini-goal you accomplish today is a moment of victory.

We can also set mini-goals spiritually. We will always be most victorious when we are in the center of God's will. When we are in God's will, we are able to see our trials from God's perspective —through the lens of His grace and truth. But what is God's will?

The apostle Paul wrote, "Rejoice always, pray continually, give thanks . . . for this is God's will" (1 Thessalonians 5:16 – 18). This is an explicit description of what God's will is. To be in the center of God's will is to be a woman who is joyful, prayerful, and thankful.

Be joyful: Intentionally look around for measures of joy each day. There is joy in simply being alive and in being redeemed by

God. Remember, joy is a choice we make, not a feeling we hope to get from our circumstances. It's good to look for the good, to celebrate it even in small ways. Doing so is a moment of victory.

Be prayerful: Focus your thoughts on God through prayer. When I was tempted with unhealthy choices, it used to trigger a pity party. Now, I turn my temptations into triggers to pray. Turning to God rather than turning to food is a moment of victory.

Be thankful: When I focus on how much weight I still need to lose, it brings me down and I start entertaining thoughts of defeat. However, when I focus on all that I'm gaining with God through this process of losing the weight, it makes me all the more determined to keep going. What is something positive you've gained during your weight loss journey so far? God's activity can be seen much more readily when we focus on what we do have rather than what we don't have.

We can't control our circumstances, but we can control our choices. Setting mini-goals physically and spiritually positions us for victory today. Indeed, *you can be victorious* even when the distance between your present reality and your desired goal seems so far apart.

Dear Lord, help me to remember that no matter how far away my goal may seem, I am most victorious when I am in the center of Your will. Today I will intentionally look for Your joy as I pray out of a thankful heart. In Jesus' name. Amen.

A Supernatural Fix

Come to me,
all you who are weary and burdened,
and I will give you rest.
(MATTHEW 11:28)

Thought for the Day: I can only find rest—fresh hope—as I stop resisting God's truths and start applying them.

Honestly, I'm tired of this being my issue! Why doesn't God step in and just supernaturally fix this?

Have you ever felt this way?

God understands what it's like to feel worn out and tired of struggling, and He hears our cry. Jesus encourages us, "Come to me, all you who are weary and burdened, and I will give you rest" (Matthew 11:28).

I used to get so frustrated when I heard this verse because I thought, "I don't want rest—I want to be restored! I want to be rid of this weight struggle once and for all!"

But the gift of rest Jesus is offering here is not a spiritual Ambien. The Greek word for this kind of rest is *anapauo* (an-ap-ow´-o) which means "of calm and patient expectation." In other words, Jesus is saying, "If you come to me, I will take your exhaustion in this area and turn it into expectation. In this place you feel hopeless, I can make you hopeful."

But how?

My friend Jennifer Rothschild does this enlightening exercise at some of her conferences. She tells the audience to imagine her writing two different words on a large chalkboard. She then speaks the letters as she draws the first word into the air ... R-E-S-T. She does the same for the second word ... R-E-S-I-S-T. Then she asks, "What's the difference?"

The difference is, of course, "I."

I can't do this. *I* can't say no. *I* can't make lasting changes. *I* don't see how the Bible can really help with this struggle.

I'm familiar with these "I" statements because I've said them myself.

We can only find *anapauo* rest—fresh hope—as we stop resisting God's truths and start applying them. Quickly skim back over the truths we've already covered in this book and find one you highlighted, got all inspired by, but haven't yet applied. Write it on a 3 x 5 card and then keep reading.

One of the assignments Jesus gives us is to take on His yoke and learn from Him (Matthew 11:29). In other words, discipline and work are necessary.

This is your part of the equation.

But after the assignment comes reassurance, "My yoke is easy and my burden is light" (Matthew 11:30). God knows where your strength ends and that is the exact point where His strength begins.

This is God's part of the equation.

I must do all I can do. Then God will do what only He can do.

My pastor, Steven Furtick, says, "You bring the natural. God will then bring the super. And that's what creates supernatural."

Dear Lord, I want to wait in calm and patient expectation today. Please take my exhaustion and turn it into expectation; take my feelings of hopelessness and give me real hope. I want to stop resisting Your truths and start applying them. I will do all that I can today, and I will wait with anticipation for all that You will do through me. In Jesus' name. Amen.

Day
23

I Need _____!

And my God will meet all your needs
according to the riches of his glory in Christ Jesus.
(PHILIPPIANS 4:19)

Thought for the Day:
Temptation is an invitation to meet my needs
outside the will of God.

Satan's very name means "one who casts something between two to cause a separation." He wants to separate us from God. One of the subtle ways he does this is to raise doubts in our mind about whether or not God will meet our needs, if God is truly enough. Satan wants us to feel alone and abandoned so that we turn to his offerings instead.

Temptation of any kind is Satan's invitation to meet our needs outside the will of God—through material things, chasing significance and approval from others, or excessive physical desires.

Often the script that plays in our head is, "I need _____ so I can be satisfied."

It's what causes a woman on a budget to set off on a spending spree. She feels the thrill of the purchase in the moment. But shame creeps in as she hides the telltale shopping bags from her family.

It's what pulls at the businesswoman to work harder and longer and refuse to build boundaries in her schedule. Always chasing that next accomplishment or that next compliment—but it's never enough.

It's what sent me on many eating sprees. The kids were loud; the house was messy; the demands of life felt beyond my control. So with great justification, I'd indulge only to end up with a bloated stomach and a deflated heart.

We expose this subtle message sold to us by Satan when we break it down to distinguish the difference between a need and a want.

All of the examples I just described are *wants*, not *needs*. Intellectually, we understand the definition of each of these words, but oh how Satan wants us to think they are one and the same.

When the difference between these two words starts to blur, we are on the road to compromising. We start justifying. And it sets us up to meet our needs outside the will of God. The abyss of discontentment invites us in and threatens to darken and distort everything in our world.

Remember, Satan is a liar. The more we fill ourselves with his distorted desires, the emptier we'll feel. The more we overspend, overwork, or overeat, the emptier we feel. Satan wants to separate you from God's best plans. He wants to separate you from God's proper provision. He wants to separate you from God's peace.

God's provision sustains life. Satan's temptation drains life.

God's provision in the short term will reap blessings in the long term. Satan's temptation in the short term will reap heartache in the long term.

God's provision satisfies the soul. Satan's temptation gratifies the flesh.

Oh sweet sister, consider these realities when making choices today. The apostle Paul writes, "My God will meet all your needs according to the riches of his glory in Christ Jesus" (Philippians 4:19). That's a promise. Trust God. Embrace truth. Live His promise.

Dear Lord, I am reminded once again of how dangerous temptations are, because they invite me to meet my needs outside of Your will. Keep me from compromising and from justifying today. I know that only Your provision sustains life and satisfies my soul. I want this truth to ring loud and clear throughout my day today. In Jesus' name. Amen.

Undistracted

But in your hearts revere [set apart]
Christ as Lord.
(1 PETER 3:15A)

Thought for the Day: Our cravings and distractions are not meant to overwhelm us. They are meant to show our ability to crave what we need the most.

When I started out on my *Made to Crave* journey, I found myself surprised by a pivotal choice. The decision that confronted me was whether or not I would "set apart" Christ as my Lord.

Many times, lesser things distracted me and even defeated me. I knew that if I was going to grow closer to God, I'd have to distance myself from distractions. At the time, the biggest issue in my life was the distraction of food. You likely chose this devotional because food is a significant distraction for you as well. However, in a time like ours, when life is complex and moves at the speed of light, we typically battle more than one distraction.

Just prior to Peter's appeal to set our hearts apart in Christ, he says, "Do not fear their threats; do not be frightened" (1 Peter 3:14).

In other words, there will be a cost to setting apart Christ as Lord. It won't be easy or comfortable. It might even make us afraid.

Maybe you've experienced the fear of failure, fear of starting strong but not reaching your goal, or fear of being scrutinized by others. I know these fears.

May I gently tuck a challenge into your soul? I want to encourage you to push past that fear today and to fast from whatever poses a distraction from God. A fast can be more than just abstaining from food. We fast whenever we remove any distraction from daily life in order to focus on God's goodness and allow him to draw us closer.

If fasting for a whole day seems like too much, then try fasting for just an hour or two. Every time you think about that desire — for food, that activity, that cigarette, or anything else that distracts you from God's goodness — use that desire as a trigger to pray. Yes, we've talked about this before, but these prayers will be more like a two-way conversation with God. Pray to Him with whispers of need, love, hope, and courage. Let His truth answer back and reassure you.

I need help.

And Jesus whispers, "[I am your] refuge and strength, an ever-present help in trouble" (Psalm 46:1).

This situation makes me afraid. Comfort me.

And Jesus whispers, "[I] will be with you; [I] will never leave you nor forsake you. Do not be afraid; do not be discouraged" (Deuteronomy 31:8).

I am tired.

And Jesus whispers, "Come to me, [when you are] weary and burdened, and I will give you rest" (Matthew 11:28).

Jesus, you feel far away and that doughnut feels very close.

And Jesus whispers, "[Nothing] will be able to separate us" (Romans 8:39).

Share your most honest thoughts in prayer by writing them out. Next to your prayers, write down one of these verses or any others that relate to your struggles. Your heart cries and His sure answers are a powerful combination.

Build on the success you have today. I assure you, dear friend, our cravings and distractions are not meant to overwhelm us. They are meant to show our ability to crave what we need the most—a soul that is no longer tangled, distracted, and hindered, because we have set apart in our hearts the lordship and love of Christ.

Dear Lord, I want to set You apart as my Lord and Savior today. Keep me from falling away. Draw me close. In Jesus' name. Amen.

The Truth Will Set You Free

"The truth will set you free."
(JOHN 8:32B)

Thought for the Day: The hard reality is, there is no magic pill and there are no quick fixes.

For years, I felt lost when it came to making healthy decisions. Honestly, I just wanted it all to be easy. I wanted the magic pill that would take off the excess pounds, tone up my saggy places without exercising, and make me feel good.

Oh, the money I wasted on the craziest infomercial schemes.

But the hard reality is, there is no magic pill and there are no quick fixes. While the focus of *Made to Crave* is not on the how-to of healthy eating, there are some researched-based truths I want to make sure we don't miss. Jesus said, "The truth will set you free" (John 8:32b). It's a principle that applies to our physical lives as well as our spiritual lives.

A key to my successful weight loss is based on the most basic of facts — more calories out than calories in. I was once confused by (and secretly allergic) to knowing the calorie count of food. But I now find it empowering to know the caloric cost of my food. I like to think of it as knowing the price tag on items I want to purchase. If I know the price, I can more easily stay within my budget. If I know the calorie count, I can more easily stay within my healthy limits.

There are many online calorie calculators and mobile apps available to help determine the calories in foods. It was enlightening for me to discover the truth about what I was eating.

Here are some other food truths from Dr. Floyd "Ski" Chilton, author of *The Gene Smart Diet*, that have helped me on my healthy eating journey:

- Women should include 25 grams of fiber per day in their diet. Some of my favorite fiber-rich foods are beans, whole grain oats, whole grain cereals, kale, almonds, apples, and fiber bars.* Fiber is a weight loss secret weapon because it helps you feel full and keeps your munchies at bay.

- Studies show that drinking 16 ounces of water first thing in the morning reduces daily caloric intake by 20 percent.

- Evenly spacing three healthy meals and two snacks throughout your day balances your blood sugar and better curbs your appetite for sugary snacks.

Many such truths and food facts available through trusted media, a doctor, or registered dietician can be eye opening to those of us who have been bound by yo-yo diets and food fads. But the most important thing to remember is that just reading this truth won't help us. We have to know it and live it.

---

*A great list of fiber rich foods can be found at http://www.genesmart.com/pages/list_of_high_fiber_foods/160.php.

The Navy Seals have a saying, "The more you sweat in training, the less you bleed in war." This statement motivates me on many levels, but I especially like how it speaks to the necessity of making healthy choices every day. What you do today matters. If you train well today, you are paving the road to victory in this battle. Be encouraged, sweet friend! Today is a new day full of opportunities to live the truth and be set free!

Dear Lord, help me to make lasting changes in how I eat.
I know You care about me and long for me to live in a place
of peace with this struggle. I believe Your truth will set me free.
In Jesus' name. Amen.

How Does Your Garden Grow?

*Commit to the LORD whatever you do,
and he will establish your plans.*

(PROVERBS 16:3)

Thought for the Day: I wanted the flowers, but not the work. Isn't that the way it is with many things in life?

One spring, I took a new route through our neighborhood and caught a glimpse of a man hard at work in his glorious flower garden. I've often looked at other people's flowers and secretly wished for my own lush display. However, the glimpse of this man with his hands digging deep into the earth brought a new revelation. He had a garden because he invested time and energy in cultivating it. He didn't wish it into being. He didn't hope it into being. He didn't just wake up one day and find that a garden of glorious blooms had miraculously popped up from the dirt.

No. He had a goal. He had a plan. He worked at it. He sacrificed for it. It took intentionality, sweat equity, determination, and consistency. And it took time and patience before he ever saw any fruit from his labor. But eventually, there was a bloom . . . and then another . . . and then another.

I saw this man's flowers and wished for my own — without a clue about all the work that had gone into producing them. I wanted the flowers, but not the work. Isn't that the way it is with many things in life? We want the results, but have no idea where to start or how much work will be required.

In addition to wishing for a garden, I also spent many years wishing for a thinner body. I had lost weight before, but I couldn't keep it off for any extended time. I was lax about actually changing what I ate, and I excused away the necessary discipline. Then I'd catch myself wishing I were thinner and making excuses about my age and metabolism, decrying the unfairness of my genetic disposition, blah, blah, blah. My changes were based more on wishful thinking than action. They were also always temporary; therefore my results were also temporary.

Consider these verses in the book of Proverbs, God's gift of wisdom and practical guidance to his people:

The plans of the diligent lead to profit as surely as haste leads to poverty. (21:5)

Commit to the LORD whatever you do, and he will establish your plans. (16:3)

When it comes to personal growth in how we care for our health, we need to move beyond wishful thinking. Consider the demands of your daily life and choose a healthy eating plan with reasonable goals based on sound medical advice. Commit your actions — your eating plan and food choices — to the Lord. Then you will reap results not just on the outside, but inside your heart where joy and peace will take root and blossom.

Dear Lord, thank You for these verses in Proverbs. I want to feed on Your truth today. I commit to turn my focus to You. Help me to plan well, work hard, and sacrifice with intention. In Jesus' name. Amen.

When the End Goal
Seems Too Hard

Make every effort to add to your faith goodness;
and to goodness, knowledge; and to knowledge, self-control;
and to self-control, perseverance.

(2 PETER 1:5 – 6)

Thought for the Day: Big things are built one brick at a time.
Victories are achieved one choice at a time.

No matter what your struggles with food may be, victory is possible today. However, most of us don't think that's true. The problem is we tend to measure only long-term success while downplaying the absolute victory found in small successes.

Remember the mini-goals we talked about?

Recently, a friend of mine called to say she'd read my blog about my healthy eating journey and as a result she walked away from indulging in a bag of M&M's. That's a victorious small success! Now, I can't say that her scale will stand up and clap and reward her with much lower numbers today. But if she builds upon this small success — choice by choice, day by day — she will see positive changes.

Though our focus in this book is satisfying life's deepest desire with God, not food, this principle applies to other struggles as well:

- If I choose not to snap at my child and instead respond with tenderness, that's a victorious small success.

- If I call a friend and offer a word of encouragement instead of shutting myself off in my loneliness, that's a victorious small success.

- If I choose to pause before responding to the rude sales clerk, thus giving her a smile instead of perpetuating her smirk, that's a victorious small success.

- If I choose to give my husband the benefit of the doubt rather than jumping to the conclusion he meant to hurt my feelings, that's a victorious small success.

Sometimes victory seems so far away because we measure it only by the end goal. And end goals can seem overwhelmingly huge, daunting, and just plain hard to reach. But if we start measuring our victories by the smaller choices we make each day, victory won't seem so impossible.

Practice this not just with your food choices, but in other areas of life as well. The more we experience the blessings of self-control, the more disciplined we'll become. We'll start to develop discipline confidence and stop buying into the lie, "This is just the way I am."

"Make every effort to add to your faith goodness; and to goodness, knowledge; and to knowledge, self-control; and to self-control, perseverance" (2 Peter 1:5 – 6). This passage reminds me that I need to add some things to my faith — I can't just say, "By faith,

I'm going to be healthy." One of those additions is self-control. And self-control starts by making one good choice.

It's amazing the chain reaction that can start in your life with just one good choice. Big things are built one brick at a time. Victories are achieved one choice at a time. A life well lived is chosen one day at a time. Oh sweet friend, you are closer than you think to victory!

Dear Lord, I want to persevere and remain strong through this healthy eating journey. I commit each small food choice to You today, knowing that I am building a path to victory one choice at a time. In Jesus' name. Amen.

Because I Am Loved

Humble yourselves, therefore,
under God's mighty hand,
that he may lift you up in due time.
(1 PETER 5:6)

Thought for the Day: Doing something in order to be loved is a trap, but doing something because I am loved is incredibly freeing.

My friend Kathrine Lee once said to me, "The first time I lost weight, I did it *so that* I'd be loved — and I gained all the weight back. This time around I'm losing weight *because* I am loved, and it's made all the difference in keeping the weight off." The truth of her statement struck me profoundly. And it applies to so much more than just weight loss.

Doing something so that we'll be loved is a trap many of us can get caught in. When I do something because I'm trying to get someone else to notice me, appreciate me, say something to build me up, or respect me more, my motives get skewed. I become very me-focused. I put unrealistic expectations on myself and the other person. And I can get stinkin' angry when I don't feel adequately noticed, appreciated, or respected.

But doing something because I am loved is incredibly freeing. Instead of looking at a relationship from the vantage point of what I stand to *gain*, I look instead at what I have the opportunity to *give*. I am God-focused and love-directed. I keep my expectations in check. And I am able to lavish on others the grace I know I so desperately need. I live free from regret, with clarity of heart, mind, and soul.

The apostle Paul wrote, "But now let me show you a way of life that is best of all. If I could speak all the languages of earth and of angels, but didn't love others, I would only be a noisy gong or a clanging cymbal" (1 Corinthians 12:31b – 13:1 NLT). And you want to know what chips away at the security of knowing I am loved? The noisy lies of the enemy. He has no love in him; therefore his voice is useless.

Are your efforts toward your goal hounded by clanging thoughts of inadequacy, fears of rejection, and hopelessness? Reject those clamorous thoughts and replace them with the love thoughts that God has sent our way through the ages:

Humble yourselves, therefore, under God's mighty hand, that he may lift you up in due time. Cast all your anxiety on him because he cares for you. Be alert and of sober mind. Your enemy the devil prowls around like a roaring lion looking for someone to devour. Resist him, standing firm in the faith, because you know that the family of believers throughout the world is undergoing the same kind of sufferings. And the God of all grace, who called you to his eternal glory in Christ, after you have suffered a little while, will himself restore you and make you strong, firm and steadfast. (1 Peter 5:6 – 10)

Isn't it interesting how much easier it is to apply Scripture when we're doing it because we're loved? Consider how this applies to the passage from 1 Peter:

> Because I am loved, I can humble myself. When I'm trying to be loved, I must build myself up to look better.
>
> Because I am loved, I can cast all my anxiety on Him. When I'm trying to be loved, I cast all my anxiety on my performance.
>
> Because I am loved, I resist Satan and stand firm in my faith. When I'm trying to be loved, I listen to Satan and stand shaky in my feelings.
>
> Because I am loved, I know God will use trials to make me stronger. When I'm trying to be loved, I wonder why God would allow trials.

Indeed, I want to pursue my goals — health and otherwise — from the vantage point of my friend Kathrine. *Because I am loved.* That's when my motives stay pure and my heart stays grounded in the comfort and assurance of God's never-changing love.

Dear Lord, I don't want my motives to get skewed during my healthy eating journey. Help me to not be me-focused in this process. I long to be God-focused because I am loved by You. Thank You. In Jesus' name. Amen.

Day
29

Conformed
or Transformed?

Do not conform to the pattern of this world,
but be transformed by the renewing of your mind.
(ROMANS 12:2A)

Thought for the Day:
I knew I couldn't be transformed
unless I refused to conform.

If you want to be a sold-out somebody for God, you have to break away from the everybody crowd.

This is not easy for a girl like me who wanted nothing more growing up than to fit in. Don't cause waves. Don't stand out. Don't stand up. Don't rock the boat in any way. Just go with the flow. But somewhere along my Christian journey, going with the flow started to bother me.

Verses like Romans 12:2a messed with my status-quo existence: "Do not conform to the pattern of this world, but be transformed by the renewing of your mind."

I knew I couldn't be transformed unless I refused to conform. Believe it or not, my getting-healthy plan is also part of my transformation — my breaking away from the everybody crowd.

Eating healthy and relying on God's strength to do it is countercultural. Your friends might not understand when you don't accept the homemade dessert even when you decline it with the utmost grace. Your kids, and even your spouse, might not understand why you no longer bring home the super-large ice cream container for family treats. The secular world will never admire your reliance on God rather than self for strength and self-control.

If your church is anything like mine, you will even be called to live counter to the typical Christian food culture in which everything served is drizzled, fried, glazed, cream filled, or chocolate covered. And while I treasure the love that's put into every act of hospitality, it's tough when your drug of choice is offered at the weekly Bible study. Really tough.

Diet-defeating tough. That's why this can't be a shortcut diet. Short-term sacrifices will lead to short-term results. I love how *The Message* paraphrase puts it: "Don't look for shortcuts to God. The market is flooded with surefire, easygoing formulas for a successful life that can be practiced in your spare time. Don't fall for that stuff, even though crowds of people do" (Matthew 7:13 – 14a MSG). Shortcuts don't work with God or with food.

Every time I make a choice I have to ask myself, "Am I being conformed, looking a lot like the crowd and staying stuck in defeat? Or, am I transformed, breaking away from the vicious cycle of defeat by courageously saying no? No more. No thank you."

Good questions to ask myself. Good questions to ponder.

This is not just a diet. This is not just another quest to get thin. This is a spiritual journey that will yield great physical benefits and subtly reject the decadent culture of this world. It is not easy, but it is good.

Dear Lord, please help me to make my healthy eating a purely spiritual journey. I want to break old habits, old addictions, and old ways for good. I need Your guidance and Your strength to help me through each day. In Jesus' name. Amen.

Day
30

Is It Sustainable?

Since we have these promises, dear friends,
let us purify ourselves from everything
that contaminates body and spirit,
perfecting holiness out of reverence for God.
(2 CORINTHIANS 7:1)

Thought for the Day: Holiness doesn't just deal with my spiritual life; it very much deals with my physical life as well.

Most people ask the same two questions when they hear about my weight loss and healthy eating plan: "How did you do it?" and "Is this something you can sustain?" In other words, they are wondering, "If I follow your advice, what will I have to give up forever?"

We often desire the long-term solution, but shy away from the actions necessary to reach our goal. Sacrificing for a season is not fun, but it is doable. However, sacrificing until we no longer desire what has been given up? Well, that just takes discipline to a whole new level. Is this kind of sacrificial discipline really sustainable?

My answer is no and yes.

No, I do not believe in our own strength we can sustain a level of discipline that requires real sacrifice for a long period of time.

However, my answer is yes if we factor in a crucial spiritual truth. Making the connection between my daily disciplines with food and my desire to pursue holiness is crucial. And holiness doesn't just deal with my spiritual life; it very much deals with my physical life as well.

It is good for God's people to be put in a place of longing so they feel a slight desperation. Only then can we be empty enough and open enough to discover the holiness we were made for. When we are stuffed full of other things and never allow ourselves to be in a place of longing, we don't recognize the deeper spiritual battle going on.

Satan wants to keep us distracted by chasing one temporary filling after another. God wants us to step back and let the emptying process have its way until we start desiring a holier life. The gap between our frail discipline and God's available strength is bridged with nothing but a simple choice on our part to pursue this holiness.

I was challenged by a pastor friend's confident statement, "God tells us to be holy. So be holy. He wouldn't have said it if it weren't possible."

This is a truth the apostle Paul affirmed when he wrote, "Since we have these promises, dear friends, let us purify ourselves from everything that contaminates body and spirit, perfecting holiness out of reverence for God" (2 Corinthians 7:1).

Moment by moment we can make the choice to live in our own strength and risk failure or to reach across the gap and grab hold of God's unwavering strength. And the beautiful thing is, the more dependent we become on God's strength, the less enamored we are with other choices.

Dear Lord, I long to experience the holiness I was made for. I want to reach across the gap and grab hold of Your strength — the unwavering strength that leads to peace and joy. In Jesus' name. Amen.

The Very Next Step
You Take

Just as you used to offer yourselves
as slaves to impurity and to ever-increasing wickedness,
so now offer yourselves as slaves to righteousness
leading to holiness.

(ROMANS 6:19)

Thought for the Day: Victory isn't a place we arrive at and then relax. Victory is when we pick something healthy over something not beneficial for us — again and again.

When I'm at my lowest emotionally, even I don't want to follow my own advice. I don't want to "be made new in the attitude of [my] mind" (Ephesians 4:23), nor do I want to "put on [my] new self, created to be like God in true righteousness and holiness" (Ephesians 4:24).

What I want to do is cry. I want to withdraw. I want to be jealous that others don't have my issues. I want to be mad at God for giving me this metabolism. And I want my very next choice to be high in calories, fried in fat, and iced with something that makes my taste buds sing.

I want victory, but I feel so weak.

This hardly sounds like someone who has conquered her food issues, right? The reality is, even when we stand on the scale and see our goal weight staring back at us, we're always just one choice away from reversing all the progress we've made.

I'm not saying victory isn't possible. It is. But victory isn't a place we arrive at and then relax. Victory is when we pick something healthy over something not beneficial for us. And we do it again. And again. We maintain our victories with each next choice.

Here's a biblical perspective from the apostle Paul:

> I put this in human terms because you are weak in your natural selves. Just as you used to offer the parts of your body in slavery to impurity and to ever-increasing wickedness, so now offer them in slavery to righteousness leading to holiness. (Romans 6:19 NIV 1984)

You see, the very next choice we make isn't really about food, weight, or even the negative feelings we carry around when we're choosing poorly. It's about whether or not we're positioning ourselves for holiness — to live the kind of God-honoring lives in which, by God's strength, sustained discipline is possible.

So how does one tap into God's strength? Certainly with prayer. Definitely through Bible reading. But there's another part to it. We tap into God's strength by practicing the gentle art of balance.

God's holy people knew there was a time to feast, a time to fast, and a time for simple daily nourishment. That's what it means to practice balance. If I understand balance, I will eat to live — not live to eat. I will enjoy nourishment, not gorge on empty calories. I will eat until satisfied, not eat to be satisfied. As Romans 6:19 says, I will make right choices that honor God and lead to holiness rather than constant indulgences that lead to defeat.

Whether the struggle is a food issue, a moral issue, an emotional issue, or a relationship issue, deep down you know when something is pulling your heart away from God. Deciding to live in a place of sustained discipline means making the choice not to view a struggle as an inevitable curse, but rather to see it as something good — something from which to learn and grow stronger. And, one good choice later, you will taste the empowerment of true balance and continue reaching forward from there.

Dear Lord, I am challenged to ponder what is pulling my heart away from You. Help me to live in a place of balance and to embrace what You have for me today. In Jesus' name. Amen.

A Deeper Purpose
for Exercise

Therefore, because of you
the heavens have withheld their dew
and the earth its crops.
(HAGGAI 1:10)

Thought for the Day: If we are really honest, we have to admit it:
we make time for what we want to make time for.

I found the most interesting story in the Old Testament about how
serious God is about people taking care of the temple entrusted
to them. Before the Holy Spirit was given to us and our bodies
became temples, the Spirit of God dwelt in such structures as a
portable, tent-like sanctuary called the tabernacle and the beautiful
temple originally built by King Solomon in Jerusalem.

During the time of the prophet Haggai, God's people had
returned from being in exile in Babylon. One of the first things
they set about to do was rebuilding the temple. They started with
great enthusiasm and wonderful intentions, but slowly slipped

back into complacency and eventually stopped their work on the temple altogether. Other things seemed higher priorities — more urgent, more appealing. Here is how Haggai describes it:

> This is what the LORD Almighty says: "These people say, 'The time has not yet come to rebuild the LORD's house.'"
>
> Then the word of the LORD came through the prophet Haggai: "Is it a time for you yourselves to be living in your paneled houses, while this house remains a ruin?"
>
> Now this is what the LORD Almighty says: "Give careful thought to your ways. You have planted much, but harvested little. You eat, but never have enough. You drink, but never have your fill. You put on clothes, but are not warm. You earn wages, only to put them in a purse with holes in it."
>
> This is what the LORD Almighty says: "Give careful thought to your ways. Go up into the mountains and bring down timber and build my house, so that I may take pleasure in it and be honored," says the LORD. (Haggai 1:2–8)

Oh, this reminds me just how divided my heart can be when it comes to taking care of my body — God's temple. Like these people, I could so easily say, "I'm not in a season where it's feasible to take care of my body. I just can't find the time between the kids, my work responsibilities, running a home, paying the bills, and all the day-to-day activities. It's just not realistic for me to exercise." But the Lord issues strong cautions to "give careful thought to [our] ways" and to make time to "build the house" so that he may be honored.

Note that God's people neglected rebuilding the temple for ten years. Each year something else seemed to be more important. That's the way exercise was for me. Year after year, something else always took precedence.

However, if I was really honest, I had to admit that I made time for what I wanted to make time for. I wasn't giving careful thought to my ways. I wasn't making a plan to exercise each day and giving that time the same priority as much more minor things. For example, I always seemed to find time to watch a favorite TV show or chat with a friend on the phone. Just the same, the Jews who returned from Babylon obviously had time to do things they really wanted to do as well. They found the time and energy to put paneling up in their own homes while ignoring the home of the Lord.

The Israelites suffered severe consequences for failing to care for the Lord's temple: "Therefore, because of you the heavens have withheld their dew and the earth its crops" (Haggai 1:10). Now, I'm not saying God will cause bad things to happen to us if we don't exercise. But there are natural consequences for not taking care of our bodies. People who don't care for their bodies now will live the consequences of those choices at some point. Whether it's more weight and less energy now or heart disease later, our choices matter both physically and spiritually. Spiritually, I feel much more weighed down by stress and problems when I'm not taking care of my body. Physically, I have less energy to serve God and more emotions to wade through when processing life.

I fully realize my temple may not be God's grandest dwelling, but I want to lift up to the Lord whatever willingness I have each day and dedicate my exercise as a gift to Him and a gift to myself.

Dear Lord, I want to care for my body in the ways I eat and in the ways I move. Help me to see the ability to exercise as a gift. I dedicate my temple to You and commit to start rebuilding it today. In Jesus' name. Amen.

Why Shouldn't I Indulge?

*I praise you because I am fearfully
and wonderfully made.*

(PSALM 139:14A)

Thought for the Day: In its proper context, eating is not the problem. God gave us food for nourishment, strength, and even celebration. The problem comes when pleasure is unrestrained.

God made you wonderful. Psalm 139 says so. You are beautiful and loved just the way you are, whether you're a size zero or a size thirty. But God loves you so much that He doesn't want you to stay in a place of defeat.

There was a time when I felt utterly defeated in the area of food and health. I knew I needed to make changes, but not because of the number on the scale or my clothing size. I knew it because of the battle that raged in my heart. I craved, I desired, I thought about, and arranged my life around food.

Yet I was a Bible teacher, a woman who loved Jesus. Why couldn't I figure this out? I had found victory in so many areas of my life, but this area alluded me. I constantly asked, "Why shouldn't I indulge?"

One day, I looked up the definition of the word *indulge*, which means to act in an unrestrained way. For me it was unrestrained eating. You see, eating in its proper context is not the problem. God gave us food for nourishment, strength, and even celebration. The problem comes when pleasure is unrestrained.

I had to get honest enough to admit that I relied on food more than I relied on God. I craved food more than I craved God. Chocolate was my comfort and deliverer. Cookies were my reward. Salty chips were my joy. Food was what I turned to in times of stress and sadness ... even in times of happiness.

I knew it was something God was challenging me to surrender to His control. Really surrender. Surrender to the point where I'd make radical changes for the sake of my spiritual health — perhaps even more than my physical health.

Part of my surrender was asking myself a really raw question. May I ask you this same question? Is it possible we love and rely on food more that we love and rely on God?

Now before you toss this book in the trash, hear me out. This question is crucial. We have to see the purpose of our struggle with food as something more than getting to wear smaller sizes and receive compliments. Shallow desires produce shallow efforts. These good things are nice, but not as appealing in the moment as a cinnamon roll, or those chips, or that brownie.

The process of getting healthy has to be about more than just losing weight and focusing on ourselves. It's not about adjusting our diets and hoping for good physical results. It's about recalibrating our souls so that we want to change for the right reasons. I discovered that pursuing a healthy eating plan was one of the most significant spiritual journeys I'd ever dared to take with God. And my hope is you're now saying the same thing!

Dear Lord, if I'm being honest with myself and You, I know sometimes I rely on food more than I rely on You. I want to recalibrate my soul and change for the right reasons. I want to see You in and through this entire process. Please be with me, Lord, each day. In Jesus' name. Amen.

Day
34

Overweight Physically and Underweight Spiritually

*"If you want to be perfect [whole], go, sell your possessions
and give to the poor, and you will have treasure in heaven.
Then come, follow me."*

(MATTHEW 19:21)

Thought for the Day: Nothing changes until we make the choice to redirect our misguided cravings to the only one capable of satisfying them.

My journey to healthy eating didn't gain traction by counting calories or obeying rules of the food pyramid. As I've said before, the process began in earnest when I admitted that, yes, I was overweight physically. But more importantly, I was underweight spiritually. I was spiritually malnourished. Tying these two issues together is what opened my eyes to see God in a whole new way.

I'm reminded of the story in the Bible where a rich young man comes to see Jesus. The man explains that he is following all the religious rules, but still feels something is missing from his pursuit of God. He asks, "What do I still lack?" Jesus responds, "If you want to be perfect [whole], go, sell your possessions and give to the poor, and you will have treasure in heaven. Then come, follow me" (Matthew 19:21).

The man then goes away sad because he won't give up the one thing that consumes him. He is so full with his riches, he can't see how undernourished his soul is. It's at this point in the biblical story that most of us start to look at all the rich people we know and think, "Well, I sure hope they get this message. Good thing I'm not rich. What a relief that Jesus doesn't ask me to sacrifice in this way." Or does He?

Jesus meant his comment for anyone who wallows in whatever abundance they have. I imagine Jesus looked straight into this man's soul and said, "I want you to give up the one thing you crave more than me."

I was like the rich young man when it came to eating. I refused healthier breakfast options, such as egg whites and fruit, while filling myself with candy-sprinkled doughnuts. I chose soda instead of water, or chips instead of carrot sticks. Even when my sugar high crashed and I complained of splitting headaches, sluggishness, and extra weight, I steadfastly refused to even consider giving up my daily brownie.

God made us capable of craving so that we'd have an unquenchable desire for more of Him, and Him alone. Nothing changes until we make the choice to redirect our misguided cravings to the only one capable of satisfying them.

Paul wrote to the Christians in Ephesus, "I keep asking that the God of our Lord Jesus Christ, the glorious Father, may give you the Spirit of wisdom and revelation, so that you may know him better" (Ephesians 1:17). I don't know about you, but to me, this one benefit of knowing God better is worth all the effort and sacrifice that a healthy eating journey requires. It's easy to feel that our struggle with food is such an unfair deal. But I encourage you to see your struggle in a new way — as a path that offers both physical and spiritual benefits.

Dear Lord, I admit that there are plenty of times that I am overweight physically and underweight spiritually. Help me to give up anything I crave more than You. I want to redirect my misguided cravings to You because You are the only one capable of satisfying them. In Jesus' name. Amen.

You Were Made for More!

I pray that the eyes of your heart may be enlightened
in order that you may know the hope to which he has called you,
the riches of his glorious inheritance in his holy people,
and his incomparably great power for us who believe.

(EPHESIANS 1:18–19A)

Thought for the Day: We were made for more! More than this failure, more than this vicious cycle of defeat, more than being ruled by our taste buds, body image, rationalizations, and guilt. We were made for victory.

More than once, I've held the latest, greatest diet book in one hand with my other hand wedged into the back pocket of my ever-tightening jeans. But the thought of taking the plunge and signing up for another diet made me want to sit down and cry. I'd return the book to the shelf, toss my head back, and sigh, "Another day, another time. I'm doing the best I can right now."

It is so tempting to quit the health struggle entirely and pretend it doesn't really matter spiritually. But it does matter — and not just for the physical or emotional setbacks. It's the denial of a fundamental spiritual truth. What is this truth?

Your parents might have told it to you when you got sassy and disrespectful: "More is expected of you. You aren't a brat, so don't act like one."

Your teacher might have told it to you when you turned in a halfhearted term paper: "You have more potential as a student than what you've shown here."

Your friends have definitely said it when your loser boyfriend dumped you: "He didn't deserve you. You're worthy of a better love than he could offer."

Today, your heavenly Father is telling you the same truth: "You were made for more!" More than this failure, more than this vicious cycle of defeat, more than being ruled by taste buds, body image, rationalizations, guilt, and shame. You were made for victory!

The apostle Paul writes:

> I pray that the eyes of your heart may be enlightened in order that you may know the hope to which he has called you, the riches of his glorious inheritance in his holy people, and his incomparably great power for us who believe. (Ephesians 1:18 – 19a)

Having the eyes of my heart enlightened with truth gives me the great power Paul is referring to here. Saying "I am made for more; I have great power" is a great script to play in our heads every time we're tempted with guilt, rationalizations, or the "I'll-do-better-tomorrow" escape clauses.

We need a power beyond our frail attempts and fragile resolve. We need strength greater than our taste buds, hormones, temptations, and our inborn female demand for chocolate. Yes, the truth of who we are and the power to live out that truth — that's what we need. So, say it out loud with me today: *I was made for more!*

Dear Lord, thank You for the truth that I am made for more.
Please help me to soak this truth in and to live it out.
Enlighten the eyes of my heart so I may believe and receive
what You have for me today. Show me a new perspective as
I seek to honor You with my choices. In Jesus' name. Amen.

I Want Legs Like Hers

A heart at peace gives life to the body,
but envy rots the bones.
(PROVERBS 14:30)

Thought for the Day: Every situation has both good and bad. When I want someone else's good, I must realize that I'm also asking for the bad that comes along with it.

If you're like me, chances are you've struggled with comparison and envy. Her stomach is flat; I've got a muffin top. Her hips are narrow; mine give new meaning to the word *curvy*. Her legs are long and lean; mine are like tree trunks.

Suddenly, all my blessings pale in comparison. What I *don't have* blinds me from seeing what I *do have*. My heart is drawn into a place of misguided assumptions and ingratitude . . . as I assume everything is great for women who possess what I don't have and I become less and less thankful for what is mine.

And here's the real kicker . . . things for the person I'm comparing myself to are almost never what they seem. If there's one lesson that living more than forty years has taught me, it's that everybody has not-so-great aspects to their lives. Whenever I get an idyllic view of someone else's life, I often say out loud, "I am not equipped to handle what they have, both good and bad."

God has had to teach me a lot about how to nip a comparison in the bud so it doesn't develop into full-blown envy and jealously. The statement, "I am not equipped to handle what they have, both good and bad," has been one of the greatest gifts God has given me. Every situation has both good and bad. When I want someone else's good, I must realize that I'm also asking for the bad that comes along with it. It's always a package deal. And usually if I'll just give something enough time to unfold, I often thank God I didn't get someone else's package.

One of the first times I came to understand this truth was in middle school when I met a beautiful girl at the children's theater in my town. We were both budding child actors cast in a Christmas play. During rehearsals, I remember seeing her long dancer's legs move in ways my stubby limbs never could. Her legs were muscular, lean, and graceful. Mine couldn't be described with any of those adjectives.

One day this girl had unusual pain in her left leg. A doctor's appointment turned into a battery of tests that turned into a hospital stay that turned into a diagnosis. Cancer. A surgery to remove a tumor turned into an amputation that turned into a complete life change. Her world was filled with words no child should ever have to know: chemotherapy, prosthetics, hair loss, and walking cane.

As a young girl, I was stunned by the whole experience. Especially because I clearly remember asking God for legs exactly like hers night after night as I watched her glide across the stage.

I was not equipped to handle what she had, both good and bad.

I don't want to paint the picture that every good thing someone else has will end with a tragedy. That's not the case. Sometimes others' good things are simply fantastic. But they are fantastic for them — not me.

I love the truth of Proverbs 14:30: "A heart at peace gives life to the body, but envy rots the bones." Sitting around wishing my legs were shapelier did nothing but discourage me and make me feel rotten. However, getting out and exercising made me come alive. It wasn't a quick fix and I still can't say I have dancer's legs, but I have peace knowing I'm doing what I can. And it is good.

Dear Lord, thank You for entrusting me only with what I have and who I am. Help me take my focus off what others have. Instead, help me make the best of what I've been given. My body is a gift. A good gift. In Jesus' name. Amen.

I Could Never Give Up That!

*The fruit of the Spirit is love, joy, peace, forbearance, kindness,
goodness, faithfulness, gentleness and self-control.*
(GALATIANS 5:22–23A)

Thought for the Day: By God's power, we are empowered. Humanly
speaking, this is impossible. But with God, everything is possible.

Self-control is hard. We don't like to deny ourselves. We don't
think it's necessary. We make excuses and declare, "That's nice
for someone else, but I could never give up _____!"
(fill in the blank: soda, sugar, cupcakes, alcohol, smoking, etc.)

If we're relying on ourselves, that excuse may be true. But there's
another level to self-control that too few of us find. Jesus says,
"Truly I tell you, it is hard for someone who is rich to enter the
kingdom of heaven ... it is easier for a camel to go through the eye
of a needle than for someone who is rich to enter the kingdom of
God" (Matthew 19:23–24).

In other words, Jesus was saying that it's hard for someone who
is satisfied with the things of this world to deny themselves. It's
hard for someone who is rich with excess to deny themselves

and be humble enough to admit, "I must give this up." When the disciples heard this teaching, they were confused until Jesus clarified, "Humanly speaking, it is impossible. But with God everything is possible" (Matthew 19:26b NLT).

We tend to think of this verse as saying, "With God, all *good* things are possible! With God, all *lavish* things are possible!" But if you study this verse in context, it actually means, "With human effort alone, it can seem impossible to deny yourself. With human effort alone, it can seem impossible to make sacrifices. With human effort alone, it can seem impossible to have self-control. But with God, all sacrificial things are possible. With God, all self-control is possible."

I believe this one vital shift in our thinking can help us shift from feeling deprived to feeling empowered. Try this little exercise at home today: Open up your fridge or your pantry and look at all the options. Say to yourself, "I'm not deprived of an unhealthy option. I'm empowered to make a healthy choice."

By God's power, we are empowered. Humanly speaking, this is impossible. But with God, everything is possible.

Rather than giving in to the foods we crave, we can have God's self-control to make completely different decisions — decisions for health, decisions for renewed energy, decisions for confidence and peace. Most importantly, decisions that honor both our bodies and God!

Dear Lord, I don't want to be caught making the statement, "I could never give up that!" Instead, I want to believe that self-control is possible because of Your strength. I want each of my decisions today to be made from a heart full of confidence and peace in You. In Jesus' name. Amen.

Day
38

I'm Not Defined
by the Numbers

*We demolish arguments and every pretension
that sets itself up against the knowledge of God,
and we take captive every thought
to make it obedient to Christ.*

(2 CORINTHIANS 10:5)

Thought for the Day: A scale is an excellent tool for determining our weight, but it's a terrible tool for determining our worth.

I was in an exercise class one day when the gal next to me leaned over and shared concerns about her sister's increasing weight. I was half listening and half straining to lift my aching legs when she quipped, "I mean, my sister now weighs like 150 pounds!" I didn't know whether to laugh out loud or keep silent, because the number that horrified her was the exact number I had seen that very morning on my scale!

I found great joy when I realized that my workout buddy's statement didn't rattle me. Just a few years ago, it would have. It would have sent me into a tailspin of crash diets and unrealistic expectations.

However, there I was, at peace in the aftermath of her thoughtless comment. I wasn't yet at my goal weight, but I was in the process of investing wisely in my health and my spiritual growth. I had been diligently filling my mind with God's truths. These principles now protected me from thoughts of condemnation, jealousy, and defeat. This is what the apostle Paul meant when he wrote, "We demolish arguments and every pretension that sets itself up against the knowledge of God, and we take captive every thought to make it obedient to Christ" (2 Corinthians 10:5).

When we are familiar with God's truth, we can challenge any comment with the questions, "Is it true? Is it beneficial? Is it necessary?" If the answer is no, then we don't open the door of our hearts. We make the choice to walk away from the comment and all the negative thoughts it could harvest if we listened to it.

My classmate's shock at her sister's weight wasn't beneficial to me. Therefore, I didn't have to internalize her comment, feed on it, and let it crush my identity. I could leave it on the gym floor and walk away because it didn't belong to me.

Right there in the gym, I desperately wanted to yell out three glorious words: "I am free!" In that moment, I experienced a small victory over an identity disorder I'd battled for a long time. This is what is true (beneficial and necessary): Jesus is the gatekeeper for the thoughts I put in my mind and the identity I allow to sink into my heart.

Lord, I want this truth to sink deeply into my heart and my mind. Help me to remember to process the thoughts and comments of others through the filter of this question: "Is this true, beneficial, and necessary?" In Jesus' name. Amen.

The Power of "I Can"

"Everything is permissible for me"
— but not everything is beneficial.
(1 CORINTHIANS 6:12A NIV 1984)

Thought for the Day: Lest we start mourning what will be lost, we must celebrate all that's being gained through our pursuit of health. "I can" instead of "I can't" is a powerful little twist of phrase for a girl feeling deprived.

Reaching my weight loss goal is a precarious place for me, a blessing entangled with a curse. The curse is the dangerous assumption that freedom now means I can return to all those things I've given up for the past months. The sacrifices, the missed treats, the deprived taste buds high on salad and low on French fries. I'm tempted to celebrate, live it up, and invite all those foods I've missed to a little welcome-home party.

Yet I can't fling open the door to all of those missed foods without welcoming back the excess calories, fat grams, cholesterol, sugars, and addictive additives. Most of these destructive guests fall under the category of junk foods. The interesting thing about these guests is that they send out little signals to our brains, begging us to party with them again and again. A welcome-home party becomes an invitation to be roommates again, which spells disaster for what we hoped might be a lifestyle change.

A chips-and-chocolate girl like me can find it hard to uninvite certain foods to the party, especially ones that have been regulars for years. It's even more difficult to acknowledge that they aren't really my friends. Some can be casual acquaintances on a very limited basis, but others need to be banished for good. Only you can determine which foods are allowed back, and which are not.

One of my favorite Scriptures for navigating this process is: "'Everything is permissible for me' — but not everything is beneficial" (1 Corinthians 6:12a NIV 1984). I quote it over and over, reminding myself that I *could* have that brownie or that cheese dip, but they wouldn't benefit me in any way. That powerful thought has helped me focus on being empowered to make a beneficial choice, rather than wallowing in feeling deprived of an unhealthy choice.

So, lest we start mourning what will be lost, we must celebrate all that's being gained through our healthy lifestyle. "I can" instead of "I can't" is a powerful little twist of phrase for a girl feeling deprived. For example:

"I can" helps me walk into a dinner party and find the conversation more appealing than the buffet.

"I can" helps me stay on the perimeter of the grocery store where the fresher, healthier selections abound and smile that I know this tidbit.

"I can" helps me reach for my water bottle and find satisfaction in its refreshment.

"I can" helps me look at the McDonald's menu and order a fruit tray without even giving a thought to the Happy Meals that used to be snacks.

"I can" reminds me to look up a restaurant's nutritional information on the Internet before going out, ensuring wiser choices.

"I can" reminds me that no food will ever taste as sweet as peace!

Dear Lord, Your Word tells us that everything is permissible, but not everything is beneficial. Remind me of this truth today when I am faced with unhealthy temptations. I can do all things with Your strength. Thank You for loving me as I struggle through this battle of a lifetime. Be with me today. In Jesus' name. Amen.

The Curse
of the Skinny Jeans

For he chose us in him before the creation
of the world to be holy and blameless in his sight.
(EPHESIANS 1:4)

Thought for the Day: Tying our happiness to food, skinny jeans, relationships, or anything else sets us up for failure. But tying our security, joy, and identity to God's love is an anchor we can cling to no matter what our circumstances may be.

Once I reached my goal weight, I thought I'd never have a bad day again. I mean really, what could possibly trouble me if I could fit into my skinny jeans? Boy, was I wrong.

A hurtful email . . . a disrespectful attitude from one of my kids . . . a missed appointment . . . a messy house . . . a stressful situation at work . . . an unexpected bill. Here I was just hours after feeling thrilled at finally being able to wear my skinny jeans, falling prey to the same topsy-turvy stuff I used to think wouldn't bother me if only I were smaller.

This is the curse of the skinny jeans.

The painful truth I've had to accept is that my body size is not tied to my happy. If I was unhappy when I was larger, I'll still be unhappy when I get smaller.

For years, I tied happiness to my circumstances and my hopes for the future. I thought, "I'll be happy when my father comes back, when I get married, when I have kids, when the economy improves, when I lose those extra pounds." But even when some of those things came true, I was still dissatisfied. Surely, there was more to me than my circumstances.

One day, I read a list of Bible verses that describe who God says I am, no matter the circumstances in my life, good or bad. I took that list of Scriptures and started to redefine my identity. It was a stark contrast to the way I'd been defining myself. I finally realized that things like my circumstances or what other people think don't define me. Instead, I could tie my happiness to the reality of who my heavenly Father says I am:

- Lysa, the forgiven child of God (Romans 3:24)
- Lysa, the set-free child of God (Romans 8:1 – 2)
- Lysa, the accepted child of God (1 Corinthians 1:2)
- Lysa, the holy child of God (1 Corinthians 1:30)
- Lysa, the made-new child of God (2 Corinthians 5:17)
- Lysa, the loved child of God (Ephesians 1:4)
- Lysa, the confident child of God (Ephesians 3:12)
- Lysa, the victorious child of God (Romans 8:37)

We were made to be free, holy, new, loved, and confident in who God made us to be. Because of this truth, we can't allow our minds to partake in anything that negates our real identity. Tying our happiness to food, skinny jeans, relationships, or anything else will only set us up for failure. But tying our security, joy, and identity to God's love is an anchor we can cling to no matter what our circumstances may be.

> *Dear Lord, I declare today that I was made to be free,*
> *holy, new, loved, and confident in who You made me to be.*
> *Protect me from anything today that challenges this truth.*
> *Help me to redefine my identity. In Jesus' name. Amen.*

Afternoon Acts
of Kindness

Teach me your way, LORD,
that I may rely on your faithfulness;
give me an undivided heart, that I may fear your name.
I will praise you, Lord my God, with all my heart;
I will glorify your name forever.

(PSALM 86:11–12)

Thought for the Day: What if I could be courageous enough to act and react like a complete person — a Jesus girl who is filled, sustained, and directed by God's joy?

I'll admit, loving incomplete people doesn't seem like the obvious path to joy. And it doesn't seem like an obvious topic to be covered in a book on getting healthy and keeping our skinny jeans in proper perspective. But stick with me here, you might be surprised.

Just the other day I was pondering some of those distressing emails I mentioned earlier, and I reached the conclusion that incomplete people are a trigger that make me want to eat. They are complicated and sensitive and messy in their reactions. They have the potential to drain my resolve and make me grumpy.

The last thing I want to do when a person throws their incompleteness in my direction is love them. I want to grab a bag of Cheetos and rationalize how much a treat is certainly in order right now. Then I want to sit on my couch and tell the air around me how much I love Cheetos and how much I dislike incomplete people.

But what if I dared in that moment to think differently? What if I could be courageous enough to act and react like a complete person—a Jesus girl who is filled, sustained, and directed by his joy? Instead of looking at this incomplete person's offense, what if I could see the hurt that surely must be behind their messy reaction?

I pause. I don't reach for the Cheetos. I don't react harshly out of my own incompleteness. I don't wallow in my thoughts of how unfair and unkind this other person is. And I choose to love instead ... taking out a piece of stationery and responding with words of grace, or crafting an email with a message of compassion.

Better yet, what if I were to do this every afternoon, even when I haven't had a run-in with an incomplete person but am just simply craving things I shouldn't eat? I've been trying this out lately and I love it. Afternoon acts of kindness are yet another unexpected but beautiful result of letting Jesus direct my healthy eating pursuits.

Each day I've been asking Jesus who in my life needs words of encouragement, and He always puts someone on my heart. So, instead of filling my afternoons with thoughts of frustration toward others or tempting thoughts about food, I am filling my afternoons with His thoughts of love toward others. And this is a great place to be, no matter if I'm wearing my skinny jeans or not.

After all, the ultimate goal of this journey isn't about making me a smaller-sized person but rather making me crave Jesus and His truths as the ultimate filler of my heart. We are to remain in this healthy perspective.

Let His thoughts be our thoughts. Remain.

Let His ways be our ways. Remain.

Let His truths go to the depths of our hearts and produce good things in our lives. Remain.

Approach this world full of fellow incomplete people with the joy of Jesus. Remain.

And see our skinny jeans as a fun reward, nothing more. Remain.

And be led forth in peace because I've kept my happy tied only to Jesus. Remain.

Dear Lord, I want to be courageous enough to act and react like a complete person today. Please help me to see areas where I need to change and grow. I desire to crave You and Your truths more than anything else because You are the ultimate filler of my heart. In Jesus' name. Amen.

Prayers Where
I Don't Speak at All

In the same way, the Spirit helps us in our weakness.
We do not know what we ought to pray for,
but the Spirit himself intercedes for us through wordless groans.
(ROMANS 8:26)

Thought for the Day: When we sit silent before God, the Spirit will intercede with perfect prayers on our behalf.

I had been going through some stinkin', rotten, horrible, no-good days and was at the absolute end of knowing what to pray. I'd slipped into a habit of praying circumstance-oriented prayers where I'd list every problem and ask God to please fix them. I even made suggestions for solutions in case my input could be useful. But nothing changed. Except my waistline and the amount of chocolate life suddenly required.

In a huff one day, I sat down to pray and had absolutely no words. None. I sat there staring blankly. I had no suggestions. I had no solutions. I had nothing but quiet tears and some chocolate smeared across my upper lip. Eventually, God broke through my worn-out heart. A thought rushed through my mind and caught me off guard: *I know you want Me to change your circumstances, Lysa. But right now I want to focus on changing you. Even perfect circumstances won't satisfy you like letting Me change the way you think.*

I didn't necessarily like what I heard during this first time of silently sitting with the Lord, but at least I felt I was connecting with God. I hadn't felt that in a long time. And so, to keep that connection, I started making it a habit to sit quietly before the Lord.

Sometimes I cried. Sometimes I sat with a bad attitude. Sometimes I sat with a heart so heavy I wasn't sure I'd be able to carry on much longer. But as I sat, I pictured God sitting there with me. He was there already, and I eventually sensed that. I experienced what the apostle Paul taught when he wrote, "In the same way, the Spirit helps us in our weakness. We do not know what we ought to pray for, but the Spirit himself intercedes for us with wordless groans" (Romans 8:26).

As I sat in silence, the Spirit interceded with perfect prayers on my behalf. I didn't have to figure out *what* to pray or *how* to pray about this situation that seemed so consuming. I just had to be still and sit with the Lord. And during those sitting times, I started to discern changes I needed to make in response to my circumstances —none of which included using food for comfort.

I think a lot of us try to get filled up with things or people. In *Becoming More Than a Good Bible Study Girl,* I talked about how I walked around for years with a little heart-shaped cup, holding it out to other people and things trying to find fulfillment. Some of us hold out our heart-shaped cup to food. Others demand that husbands love us in ways that right our wrongs and fill up our insecurities. Sometimes we expect our kids to be successful so that we look good and have our worth validated by their accomplishments. Or we overspend our budget on an outfit we just have to have.

Whatever it is, if we are really going to make lasting changes, we have to empty ourselves of the lie that other people or things can ever fill our hearts to the full. Then we have to deliberately and intentionally fill up on God's truths and stand secure in His love.

The more I fill myself up with the truths of God's love, the less I find myself pulling out that little heart-shaped cup. I have to mentally replace the lies with truth to remind myself of just how filling God's love really is.

Dear Lord, I often don't have words to pray. Remind me that as I'm silent before You, the Spirit intercedes for me. Please protect me from the lies that seem to creep into my mind at a moment's notice. Help me today, Lord, to keep my mind fixed on You. In Jesus' name. Amen.

A Soul Longing to Be Filled

I spread out my hands to you;
I thirst for you like a parched land.

(PSALM 143:6)

Thought for the Day: When the desire for treats is triggered by
difficult emotions, it's not really a desire for treats. It's a thinly veiled
attempt at self-medication.

A starved soul is like the vacuum cleaner my mother used when
I was a child. It had a long metal tube that ravenously sucked up
anything and everything set before it. It sucked up dust bunnies
with the same furor as a $10 bill. I know that one from experience.

Our souls have the same ravenous intensity as my mother's
vacuum cleaner; that's how God created us — with a longing to be
filled. It's a longing God instilled to draw us into deep intimacy
with Him. The psalmist expresses this longing as an intense thirst:

> As the deer pants for streams of water, so my soul pants for you,
> my God. My soul thirsts for God, for the living God. When can
> I go and meet with God? (Psalm 42:1–2)

I spread out my hands to you; I thirst for you like a parched land. (Psalm 143:6)

Indeed, our souls are thirsty and ravenous vacuums. If we fail to understand how to fill our souls with spiritual nourishment, we will forever be triggered to numb our longings with other temporary physical pleasures. When those pleasures are food, the resulting behavior is what we often hear referred to as "emotional eating." But this issue is bigger than emotions; it's really about spiritual deprivation.

My boyfriend breaks up with me. I want a tub of ice cream.

That big business deal falls through. I'll take the super-sized fries, please.

I don't feel pretty. I need some chocolate to soothe and delight me.

My kids are driving me crazy. I deserve a piece of cake. I deserve three pieces.

I hate cleaning my house. When I'm done I'll treat myself to as many chips as I want.

It's my birthday and I don't really think anyone cares. I'll just eat my way into happiness or numbness.

Same difference, right?

I hardly think it ironic that I'm struggling even as I write these words. There's a situation in my life that has wormed its way straight to the most vulnerable of places in my heart. This situation has made me feel hurt and rejected. Years ago a little crack in my strong resolve was created by the extreme rejection of my biological father. And while I've found amazing victory in understanding I'm no longer a child of a broken parent but rather a child of God, revisiting rejection is never fun.

I'm not saying we shouldn't allow ourselves the occasional treat. We should. But I've realized when the desire for treats is triggered by difficult emotions, it's not really a desire for treats. It's a thinly veiled attempt at self-medication. And self-medicating with food even once triggers vicious cycles I must avoid.

When difficult emotions come, I must realize stuffing myself with food only serves to compound the bad feelings later. What I need in this moment is to do something good, positive, and healthy for myself. Take a walk, read an inspirational book, write an encouraging note to a friend, memorize an uplifting verse, or play some of my favorite praise songs really loudly while driving through the country. This is just a start of my list of positive things to do that refresh me. What would be on your list? What refreshes, refuels, and refills your soul?

Dear Lord, I have connected emotional emptiness with a desire for more food. Please help me to deal with these triggers so I can recognize them for what they are and put them to rest. In Jesus' name. Amen.

The Weekly Weigh-In

You have filled my heart with greater joy
than when their grain and new wine abound.
(PSALM 4:7 NIV 1984)

Thought for the Day: It's easy to do the right things when we see immediate results. But sometimes it pleases God more to do the right thing even when the results are not so immediate.

While I no longer need to go to my nutritionist for a weekly weigh-in, I thought you might enjoy reading something I wrote in the midst of my weight loss journey . . .

So yesterday I went for my weekly weigh-in with my nutritionist. I approach this time with her each week with mixed feelings.

If her scale is kind, it makes me want to throw my arms around her and call her my BFF.

If her scale is cranky, it makes me want to throw my hands on my hips in protest and tell her how unfair it is that I have to stand on that scale fully clothed. Not that the alternative is really an option; I'm just saying. Those clothes weigh something. And I don't want that something making my numbers go up.

When I weigh at home, I don't even wear a ponytail holder. Not kidding.

So.

Her scale was cranky this week. And I didn't even have one lick of the redneck surprise served at the family get-together. (It's a desert involving chocolate and ice cream, need I say more?) Not one lick.

How fair is that?

I was lamenting via text messages with my ever-wise friend and exercise partner, Holly, and this is our dialogue after my initial whine and complaint:

HOLLY: What matters most is that you are being obedient and using discipline as a means of worship to Him ... the numbers will fall as they may.

LYSA: Yes, but I like it much better when the numbers fall on the downward side.

HOLLY: They will fall. Trust me.

LYSA: I know, but it sure does make my worship more joyful when I know I am eating correctly, and I'm actually losing weight. It's a bummer to be stuck for two weeks (and I didn't even eat any of that stinking redneck surprise — I didn't type that, but I sure was thinking it).

HOLLY: You ARE doing it correctly ... you know that. It takes perseverance. We wouldn't want it to be easy, would we? Be rare.

LYSA: (no comment ... I couldn't rub my toes that just got stepped on in a good way and type at the same time.)

HOLLY: And remember the worship is about HIM, not you. THAT will make you joyful.

LYSA: You are so right—thanks for the reminder. I'm still happy when I see the numbers go down though. That's rare too!

And so goes another day in the life of this healthy-eating pursuit. I guess my next spiritual challenge is to be more motivated by the reality that I'm *doing* the right thing rather than *seeing* the right thing on the scale.

What a great spiritual lesson for more than just healthy eating.

It's easy to do the right things when we see immediate results. But sometimes I think it pleases God more for his girls to do the right thing even when the results are not so immediate.

Holly is right. My focus must be on eating healthy as an act of worship to God, not the numbers on the scale.

As the psalm writer said, "You have filled my heart with greater joy than when their new grain and new wine and redneck surprise abound."

I got special permission to add in that last part.

Dear Lord, I want to be motivated by the reality of doing the right thing more than seeing the right thing on the scale. But this is so difficult at times, Lord, it really is. My desire is to worship You and please You through this journey more than anything else. I ask for Your strength to continue. In Jesus' name. Amen.

Knowing but Not Applying

Surely you desire truth in the inner parts;
you teach me wisdom in the inmost place.
(PSALM 51:6 NIV 1984)

Thought for the Day:
There is a big difference between ingesting and digesting.

It wasn't uncommon for me a few years back to read a diet book while mindlessly munching on chips. Or, curling up on the couch to watch *The Biggest Loser* with a bowlful of ice cream.

There is a big difference between ingesting and digesting.

Just taking in the inspiration of truth but never being transformed by it will lead you down a dangerous path of doubt. Doubting yourself. Doubting God. Doubting the effectiveness of truth.

And what a tragedy that is.

I should know. Too many times, I've been one to ingest without digesting: reading truth, but not applying it; liking a message I hear at church, but not living it; knowing what I must do to experience life change, but never putting it into action; taking in knowledge, but never letting it make a difference in my life.

Sweet sister, can we honestly admit together that we've all been there? And then can we agree together that we don't have to stay there?

When I initially posted these thoughts on my blog, I asked, "What is a healthy choice you have made recently or could make part of your life today?" The answers inspired me.

I am going to go grocery shopping and fill my fridge and cabinets with healthy options. It's amazing how much more healthy I eat when I plan to do so in advance. I'm actually excited about this!

My healthy choices are that I added fresh fruit and vegetables to my eating habits. I have also increased my water intake. It paid off I lost 1.6 pounds this last week. Woo hoo! Healthier choices do make a difference.

My healthy choice for today was to get in another Zumba class this week!

My healthy choice for today is only eating when I'm truly hungry and not just "emotionally" hungry! Thanks for the article today. I needed the extra motivation.

I'm going to go run today. I want my body to get to the place where it craves exercise on a daily basis. Right now I have to work hard to motivate myself to get moving.

I have started using the treadmill. Today was the farthest I've ever gone — 2.5 miles at 3.2 mph.

I keep saying, "I know what to do; it's just *doing* it that's the problem." I am eliminating sugar today. I have done this for almost two weeks, but yesterday chose to go my own way (ignoring all the principles I've learned and have been applying). So I'm steering back to the path He's having me walk. Thank You, Lord. I will digest, not just ingest!

What is a healthy truth you've been ingesting but not digesting? Why not let it sink deep? Start with just one thing. Maybe it's a physical choice, like drinking enough water. Or, maybe it's a spiritual choice, like believing you were made for more than this vicious cycle of defeat. Whatever it is, make progress there. Ingest that truth. Then digest it until it becomes part of who you are.

Dear Lord, I am inundated with information about how You want me to live. I hear Your truths at church, on the radio, in conversations with friends, when I read my Bible, and during Bible studies. These are all good things, but sometimes it feels overwhelming. Still, I want to do better. Forgive me for ingesting, not digesting Your truths. Help me to digest at least one truth a day so that I start living Your messages instead of just hearing them. In Jesus' name. Amen.

Frustrated with God

But seek first his kingdom and his righteousness,
and all these things will be given to you as well.
(MATTHEW 6:33)

Thought for the Day: God's goal isn't for us to be skinny. God's goal is for us to be healthy—spiritually and physically.

If God is so big and mighty and able, why doesn't God just fix us instantly? Have you ever wrestled with this question? Many of us have.

Recently, a blog reader typed out this gut-honest response in the midst of reading *Made to Crave*:

Okay, I know it sounds awful to say this, but I'm frustrated with God. Why can't He just make it impossible for me to make wrong choices with my eating? Why doesn't He help me? Can't He just be bold and say, "Don't eat that!" Or better yet, why doesn't He just fix my weight issues? Sometimes it's so hard to feel like He really cares.

Oh sister, I understand. On the surface it does seem like the kindest thing for God to do would be to fix us instantly. Or at least give us taste buds that sing when we eat raw veggies but gag when we eat cupcakes. Right?

But here's the absolute truth about God. He is kind. He is loving. He is compassionate. And He's not giving us quick fixes. This leads me to believe the quick fixes aren't the kind, loving, compassionate answers we think them to be.

You see, God's goal isn't for us to be skinny. God's goal is for us to be healthy — spiritually and physically.

My weight issues were an external indication of an internal situation. God wants me to address the internal issue of craving food more than I crave Him. If I don't address the root of this issue, I will never be satisfied. Even in a skinny body, I would be restless, depressed, anxious, unhappy, and unsatisfied if my soul isn't craving God most.

Consider this comment from another blog reader: "Please don't mistake skinny for happy. I tackled my food issues by redirecting my cravings for food to craving attention and affirmation from others. I am thin, but I am not satisfied."

As I said, God wants us to learn to crave Him most of all. More than food. More than affirmation from others. More than material possessions. More than anything else this world has to offer.

Jesus tells us, "Seek first his kingdom and his righteousness, and all these things will be given to you as well" (Matthew 6:33). Interestingly enough, when I looked up the word *seek* in the original Greek, I found the word *zeteo* (dzay-teh´-o), which means "to crave." Consider this expression of craving: "How lovely is your dwelling place, LORD Almighty! My soul yearns, even faints, for the courts of the LORD; my heart and my flesh cry out for the living God" (Psalm 84:1 – 2).

When tempted to stray from my healthy eating commitments, I have to honestly ask myself, "Am I eating this because I need food? Or am I trying to fill a craving for God in my soul?" Food can fill my stomach but never ease the ache for God in my soul.

And that's precisely the reason I now thank God for allowing me to go through this struggle. If I had never had external indications of my internal situation, I would have missed this profound and life-changing discovery.

Dear Lord, I never thought I'd say this about my weight struggles, but thank You. Thank You for giving me an external indication that forces me to look at my internal situation. I want to want You more than anything else. In Jesus' name. Amen.

Weak Places,
Strong Places

The LORD is my rock, my fortress and my deliverer;
my God is my rock, in whom I take refuge.

(PSALM 18:2A)

Thought for the Day: Even the smallest drop of God's strength is more than enough to cover our frailties, our shortcomings, the places where we deem ourselves weak.

We all have them. Weak places. Places inside us that make us wonder if we'll ever get it together like the together people. Places that make us feel less than. Less than victorious. Less than a conqueror. Less than strong.

My weak places frustrate me. I just resolved to do better three weeks ago and already I'm slipping in a couple of places. And yet I refuse to resign myself to the thought that I can't ever change.

With the power of Christ, all things can be made new. All broken things are subject to restoration. But sometimes I get so tired of trying and I just feel weak. Can you relate?

What is your weak place? A food issue that rages even though you just signed up for that new diet program? A money situation that seems impossible? A temper that flares? An insecurity that stings?

Let me breathe a little life into your weakness today. Whatever it is, however large it may loom ...

You don't have to have all the answers. You don't have to make suggestions to God. It's okay to be so tired of your weak places that you run out of words to pray.

And listen to the beautiful verses written to us Jesus girls about weak places:

> There is now no condemnation for those who are in Christ Jesus. (Romans 8:1)

> You, however, are controlled not by the sinful nature but by the Spirit. (Romans 8:9a NIV 1984)

> If God is for us, who can be against us? (Romans 8:31b)

> No, in all these things we are more than conquerors through him who loved us. (Romans 8:37)

Maybe we need to sit still for just a moment or two today. Quiet, without the weight of condemnation or the swirl of trying to figure things out. Quiet, with nothing but the absolute assurance the Spirit helps us in our weakness.

The Spirit knows what to pray. He understands our weak places. There is a purpose to this weak place. Though it doesn't feel good now, things will be worked out in a way that good will come from it (Romans 8:28).

In that quiet stillness, while the Spirit prays for us and we just simply soak in truth, there will be a flicker of light. A slight trickle of hope. A grace so unimaginable, we'll feel His power overshadowing our weakness. Even the smallest drop of God's strength is more than enough to cover our frailties, our shortcomings, the places where we deem ourselves weak.

And we'll reject that word.

We aren't weak.

We are dependent. Dependent on the only one powerful enough to help us. The only one sufficient enough to cover us in grace throughout the process.

Our relationships may not be sufficient. Our circumstances may not be sufficient. Our finances may not be sufficient. Our willpower may not be sufficient. Our confidence may not be sufficient. But God is and has been and forever will be. He says, "My grace is sufficient for you, for my power is made perfect in weakness" (2 Corinthians 12:9a).

Instead of wallowing in my weak place, I will let the Spirit reveal the one positive step I can take today. I will wash away the condemnation with the warmth of His grace. I will receive His power. And I will rename the weakness my strong place. "For when I am weak, then I am strong" (2 Corinthians 12:10b).

Dear Lord, I am weak without You. Please help me to have enough faith to get through the next challenging situation I will face today. And then enough faith for the next. Thank You for Your love, grace, mercy, and the sacrifice You made on the cross for me. In Jesus' name. Amen.

Day 48

Desperation
Breeds Defeat

No temptation has overtaken you
except what is common to mankind. And God is faithful;
he will not let you be tempted beyond what you can bear. . . .
He will also provide a way out so that you can endure it.

(1 CORINTHIANS 10:13)

Thought for the Day: Desperation does indeed breed defeat. But God promises answers for desperate situations.

I was walking through the airport when an incredible aroma suddenly grabbed my attention and taunted, *Do you know how happy I can make you?* A candy shop had just made a fresh batch of nutty, caramel popcorn.

There's nothing wrong with caramel popcorn except that it definitely wasn't on the healthy eating plan I'd committed to. I felt my knees get weak because I love caramel popcorn. I started to rationalize buying this special treat, thinking, "I can't get this at home, and I'll take half home to my kids. What harm will a little caramel popcorn do?" I felt an extreme gravitational pull straight to the object of my desire.

The only thing that stopped me was redirecting my thoughts away from the popcorn and onto a new truth God had been teaching me: desperation breeds defeat. This truth was the perfect match for my temptation and helped me walk away.

The book of Genesis tells an interesting story about twin brothers who illustrate this point. The elder son, Esau, was favored by his father, Isaac, because of his prowess as a hunter. In contrast, the younger son, Jacob, was a quiet homebody.

One day, Esau returned home from an unsuccessful hunting trip totally famished and demanded some stew from his brother. "I'll give you food," agreed Jacob, "but first, trade me your birthright."

"Okay," Esau replied, "I'm so hungry, I'm about to die." So Esau traded the honors due to him as the firstborn son for a simple meal of stew.

On first glance, it's easy to ridicule Esau's decision. I cannot imagine selling my whole birthright for a pot of soup. But I had to look at my own life and ask, "What great thing have I traded for so little in return? How often do I trade healthy food for junk food? What temporary pleasure have I craved so much that I gave up lasting victory?"

Desperation does indeed breed defeat. But God promises answers for desperate situations. The "way out" that God provides is the ability to decide in advance what I will and will not eat each day.

I plan my meals right after breakfast when I'm feeling full and satisfied. The absolute worst time for me to decide what I'm going to eat is when I've waited until I'm depleted and feeling hungry. So I prepare a healthy snack to have on hand or keep in my purse.

When I'm unprepared or I've rushed through a proper meal, my stomach screams for something quick. And quick options usually come in a variety of unhealthy temptations, just as I experienced at the airport. However, that day I had decided ahead of time that I would keep an apple in my purse for a snack, rather than trade my healthy progress for something like caramel popcorn.

If we purposely think and plan before we eat, we'll be better able to see the "way out" that God promises when we are tempted —and to keep our cravings centered on God alone.

Dear Lord, I acknowledge that I need You. I need You in my times of desperation, and I also need You in times of jubilation. Help me to think ahead so I won't be weak when I am faced with temptation. In Jesus' name. Amen.

Ignorance Isn't Bliss

So, as the Holy Spirit says:
"Today, if you hear his voice,
do not harden your hearts."
(HEBREWS 3:7 – 8A)

Thought for the Day: I can't keep driving through the dangerous intersection of reality and think it won't ever affect me.

My pastor made a statement recently we've all heard: Over 50 percent of marriages are ending in divorce today. But then he added a question that really made me think. "If you knew there was an intersection where 50 percent of the people who drove through it were killed, wouldn't you find a different route home?"

I sat back. This question snagged on the edge of my mind and lingered. Yes, certainly it applies to the marriage statistic, but it applies to my food issues as well.

Here are the statistics:*

---

*Source: Dr. Ski Chilton: (http://www.genesmart.com/pages/inflammation/69.php).

- Current figures from the Centers for Disease Control and Prevention (CDC) put the prevalence of obesity among adults at about 66 percent.

- Inflammatory diseases such as cardiovascular disease, diabetes, cancer, arthritis, asthma, allergies, depression, and Alzheimer's are increasing at dramatic rates.

- Alarming trends in obesity and inflammatory diseases are significant contributors to our nation's escalating health care costs. Health care accounts for $1 in every $6 spent in the United States.

- Nearly 24 million Americans — 8 percent of the population — have diabetes, according to statistics released by the CDC in 2008. Even more shocking have been the data from individual states. In 1991, only nine states had diabetes rates of 7 to 8 percent, with none higher. By 2001, 43 states had diabetes rates of at least 7 to 8 percent, with Mississippi, Alabama, and Florida exceeding 10 percent. Estimates are that by 2025, the number of Americans with the disease will be close to 50 million.

- Arthritis and joint disease affect 43 million people in the United States, almost 20 percent of the population. This number is expected to surpass 60 million by 2020.

So, here's where I had to stop denying issues and start paying attention to the dangerous intersection between my choices and my health. My medical chart was labeled "obese." I know — I was shocked that only thirty pounds overweight had pushed me into the obese category. But what's important to remember is I had a high body fat to lean tissue ratio. I knew my poor food choices were only making things worse. My body felt the pain of carrying too much weight. And my defeated spirit felt the weight of carrying too much pain. Yet, for years, I refused to find another way. A healthy way. A better way home.

"So, as the Holy Spirit says: 'Today, if you hear his voice, do not harden your hearts'" (Hebrews 3:7–8a). This verse refers to the Old Testament story of the Israelites becoming hard-hearted by disobeying God and refusing to conquer the Promised Land. The Greek word for "hear" in this verse is *akouoa* (ak-oo´-o), meaning "to attend to, consider what is or has been said." The Greek word for "harden" is *skleruno* (sklay-roo´-no), meaning "to become obstinate or stubborn." It sure does make me stop and consider my own refusals to conquer my issues and embrace a better, healthier future. I can't be stubborn and refuse to attend to and consider all that I know God has been speaking to me about this issue.

I can't ignore the statistics. I can't keep driving through the dangerous intersection of reality and think it won't ever affect me. Truly, with this issue ignorance is anything but bliss. And sometimes it's just good to face the gut-honest reality.

I know this isn't the most fun devotion in this book. So keep reading in Hebrews until you reach this hopeful promise:

> For we do not have a high priest who is unable to empathize with our weaknesses, but we have one who has been tempted in every way, just as we are — yet he did not sin. Let us then approach God's throne of grace with confidence, so that we may receive mercy and find grace to help us in our time of need. (Hebrews 4:15–16)

It's so comforting to know Jesus felt what I sometimes feel — He can empathize with me. And because He does, I can face my issues and not feel so alone. I can be gut-honest with myself and with Jesus and say, "Help me find a better route home."

Dear Lord, I can't ignore the statistics any longer. Reveal to me the hope that can only come from You. I need Your hope to get through today. I need to step up and consider the facts. I long to pursue a healthier lifestyle — both physically and spiritually. In Jesus' name. Amen.

Don't Eat Your Way Out of the Pit

Three times a day [Daniel] got down on his knees and prayed,
giving thanks to his God, just as he had done before.

(DANIEL 6:10B)

Thought for the Day: Each thing for which I verbalize my thankfulness is like a stepping-stone out of the pit.

Have you ever been in a pit? Yesterday, I was. And you know what pits make me feel besides frustrated and down? Hungry.

Usually my pit comes when circumstances roll into my life that I can't control. Circumstances that are beyond my control make me want to find comfort in things I *can* control. And eating sure does feel like an easy way to get comfort.

But in these situations, what feels comforting going into my mouth often doesn't settle well with my heart.

Overindulging in junk food makes me feel guilty. And once guilt joins me in my pit, it only compounds my issues. So, if we can't eat our way out of a pit with junk food, what can we do?

If I'm truly hungry, I grab a healthy option. Then, I intentionally look for something for which to be thankful and get my mouth busy praising God.

Even though I may not feel like praising God in the midst of my pit, something starts to shift in my heart and in my attitude when I see blessings in the midst of burdens. Each thing for which I verbalize my thankfulness is like a stepping-stone out of the pit.

And this isn't just my idea. It's biblical. Look what happened when Daniel took this approach to the pit he found himself in.

Daniel had just learned that anyone caught praying to any god besides King Darius would be thrown into the lions' den. That's a serious pit! But Daniel's reaction is amazing.

He went home, threw open his windows, and prayed anyway. I'm not thinking he did this because he felt good. I'm imagining he felt like anyone would feel in overwhelming circumstances. But he rose above his feelings to make a courageous choice.

And do you know what he chose to pray?

"God, save me!"

"God, it's not fair!"

"God, this is too much!"

"God, smite my enemies and wipe them out!"

"God, you know I can't handle this without extreme doses of chocolate!"

No. None of the above.

What Daniel prayed is a powerful lesson for me.

Daniel prayed, *Thank You, God.* "Three times a day he got down on his knees and prayed, giving thanks to his God, just as he had done before" (Daniel 6:10b).

Since Daniel's response is so opposite of the way most of us would react, it makes me stop and ponder. Our initial responses are usually a by-product of the rituals we've established in our lives. Daniel had made it his habit to be thankful. Therefore, who God is and what God provides was front and center in Daniel's heart —even in the midst of heartbreak.

I am so challenged and inspired by this. Where do I run when life presses in on me? On whom or on what am I really dependent? Do I have a habit of inviting guilt to join me in my pit? What might happen if I stopped grabbing for comfort and instead embraced the perspective change of thanksgiving?

Yes, life will be full of pits. But that doesn't mean I have to be a pit dweller or a pit eater.

Dear Lord, I know it is normal for us to sometimes find ourselves in a pit. But we don't have to stay there and we don't have to try to eat our way out. Thank You for providing Your timeless Word to point to the way, the truth, and the life. In Jesus' name. Amen.

I Am More than the Sum Total of My Taste Buds

Those who live according to the flesh
have their minds set on what the flesh desires;
but those who live in accordance with the Spirit
have their minds set on what the Spirit desires.

(ROMANS 8:5)

Thought for the Day: "Taste buds, you aren't the boss of me!" Whatever my physical struggle, I can't believe the lie that victory isn't possible for me. It is.

One thing that helped me so much in my physical struggle with unhealthy eating was realizing I'm more than a sum total of my taste buds. And it really is possible to boss my taste buds around!

When I was a little girl, I was never one who liked to be bossed around. As a matter of fact, I distinctly remember wondering who was the boss of all the bosses? That's who I wanted to be. So, in my little girl brain, I reasoned the President of the United States was the job for me. I'd sit behind a big desk and get paid to remind people, "You're not the boss of me! It's my way or the highway."

I'm not proud of my childish attitude, which has certainly been humbled since then. But I sure do wish I could bottle up some of that tenacity when it comes to eating healthy. I'd do well to put my hands on my hips and remind my taste buds, "You're not the boss of me. It's my way or the highway!"

My heart doesn't crave that candy bar. My arms don't desire those French fries. My brain doesn't need those chips. My soul doesn't cry out for that milkshake. And my heinie certainly doesn't want that cheesecake. Only my taste buds want that. So, I must let my arms, brain, heart, soul, heinie, and the whole of who I am boss my taste buds around.

But this won't be easy if I don't come up with an arsenal of yummy-tasting foods that are healthy. God gave me taste buds, which leads me to believe I am supposed to enjoy eating. It's not just a function of sustaining life. Eating is to be enjoyed. But eating was never supposed to sabotage my life either. *Deep fried, smothered and covered, drizzled and drenched, salted and seasoned beyond reason* are all words that speak of the sabotage to which I'm referring.

Fresh, whole, organic, raw, and *natural* are all words that speak of the life sustenance we can learn to enjoy. Some of my favorite new healthy options are raw veggies dipped in hummus, strawberries and other fresh-cut fruits sprinkled with Stevia, and oatmeal mixed with berries and nuts.

Just a few years ago I would have turned my nose up at those healthy options and reached for a doughnut. But that's where bossing my taste buds has come into play. I've trained myself to enjoy healthy options and you know what amazes me? I now crave what I've trained myself to enjoy.

Amazing. I now happily and willingly choose fruit over fried every time. I guess a little of that childish sass isn't so bad after all. You might want to try it: "Taste buds, you aren't the boss of me!"

Dear Lord, thank You for loving me despite my struggles.
You know me and love me every day and I thank You for that.
Help me to change my food cravings. I desire to eat healthy.
Help me to be victorious today. I know I was made for more
than what my taste buds tell me. In Jesus' name. Amen.

One or Two Verses a Day

Alarmed, Jehoshaphat resolved
to inquire of the LORD.
(2 CHRONICLES 20:3A)

Thought for the Day: God's words are so rich, so penetrating, and so intentionally placed, I don't want to rush past a powerful few in an effort to get through a whole chapter.

Have you ever felt pressure to read more in order to have a better quiet time?

I don't think more always equals better.

Sometimes, truly, less is more.

For example, one of the messages I'm speaking at conferences right now is about King Jehoshaphat (2 Chronicles 20). I love the first three words of verse 3, "Alarmed, Jehoshaphat resolved ..." Right within those three words is a message that will preach—and should preach—to me all day long.

A message in three words, you ask?

Yes, ma'am.

I love how Jehoshaphat's name is book-ended in two opposite words.

"Alarmed" is how he was feeling.

"Resolved" is how he responded to his situation despite his feeling.

Jehoshaphat had just found out that three countries were banding together to fight against his smaller army. Yes, he should have felt alarmed. But what inspires me is his ability not to react out of his alarm. He stayed resolved, "resolved to inquire of the LORD." In other words, his feelings were an appropriate *indicator* of what he was facing but not a *dictator* for his reaction.

Here's the message that preaches to me: "My feelings should be an indicator of my situation but never a dictator of my reaction."

This applies to my eating and weight struggles. It applies to my relationship struggles. It applies to so many struggles.

I want to be resolved — resolved to inquire of the Lord. So, though my quiet time might consist of just three words, pondering how to be resolved will linger in my thoughts all day. And it will surely change my reactions, my words, and my thoughts.

How might the same thing happen when you unearth some of God's treasures tucked within just a few of His words? I've unearthed a lot of verses that relate to satisfying our deepest desire with God, not food. But there are more to be discovered. Find them! And then relate them to what you are facing today. Here are some great verses to get you started:

> I lift up my eyes to the mountains — where does my help come from? My help comes from the LORD, the Maker of heaven and earth. (Psalm 121:1 – 2)

Jesus replied, "You do not realize now what I am doing, but later you will understand." (John 13:7)

In addition to all this, take up the shield of faith, with which you can extinguish all the flaming arrows of the evil one. (Ephesians 6:16)

They seldom reflect on the days of their life, because God keeps them occupied with gladness of heart. (Ecclesiastes 5:20)

Do not be afraid of them; the LORD your God himself will fight for you. (Deuteronomy 3:22)

By faith Noah, when warned about things not yet seen, in holy fear built an ark to save his family. (Hebrews 11:7a)

For it is God who works in you to will and to act in order to fulfill his good purpose. (Philippians 2:13)

What treasures did you discover among these Scriptures? Write them down and consider the individual meaning of each and the collective meaning of the statement as a whole. Then spend the day pondering the personal message God has for you.

Dear Lord, I love Your Word. I love the simple but very profound verses listed on this page. Help me to see You in each word. Help me to understand Your truth and to live it out today. I am Your child and I am dearly loved. Thank You, Lord. In Jesus' name. Amen.

Day
53

The Courageous Choice

Be on your guard; stand firm in the faith;
be courageous; be strong.
(1 CORINTHIANS 16:13)

Thought for the Day: Making a courageous choice means walking on the path of discipline in the area of our food choices. It's coming to the realization that changes need to be made — and making those changes in the quietness of the pantry, when no one else is looking.

I recently had the most interesting conversation with a friend who lives in Hollywood. This person lives in the midst of glitz, glamour, and extreme excess. She lives in that world, but refuses to live like that world. She is determined to teach her kids something rare ... the courageous choice. And while Hollywood seems far away from me and my life situations, the courageous choice is something we all face no matter where we live and what issues we're facing.

Throughout this conversation I kept thinking about our courageous choices with food.

You see, there are two kinds of courage. There's the courageous act, which is what makes our heart beat fast when the knight fights the dragon or the firefighter rushes into the burning building. These are extreme events most of us won't ever face. And because most of us aren't put in positions to participate in a courageous act, we don't necessarily think of ourselves as courageous.

But there's a second kind of courage that is widely available but not widely embraced. It's the courageous choice. This is the decision to do the right thing even when it's unpopular, uncelebrated, and probably even unnoticed.

The right thing is to make healthier choices for ourselves. The right thing is to satisfy our deepest needs with God, not food. It's the choice to walk willingly on the path of discipline in the area of our food choices. It's coming to the realization that changes need to be made — and making those changes in the quietness of the pantry, when no one else is looking.

It's respecting ourselves enough to be courageous for us.

It is possible to quiet the battle in your mind. It is possible to make the courageous choice. It is possible to stand in that pantry and declare you were made to consume food but food was never meant to consume you.

It is possible to consume only that which will add to your health and not take away from it. It is possible.

So make that choice. And then make it again. And then make it again.

You are courageous. Now go out and prove it to yourself.

Dear Lord, I acknowledge that I need Your divine help with each choice I make every day. I don't ever want to step outside Your will and direction for my life. I am courageous only with You, in You, and through You. Please help me to embrace Your courageous choices for me. In Jesus' name. Amen.

Naysayers

Therefore, my dear brothers and sisters, stand firm.
Let nothing move you.
Always give yourselves fully to the work of the Lord,
because you know that your labor
in the Lord is not in vain.

(1 CORINTHIANS 15:58)

Thought for the Day: As Jesus girls, we can't let the naysayers in life drown out our excitement, our calling, and our assignments from Jesus. We have to shut off the source and stop the flow of negativity in our life.

I bet there has been a time or two in your life when you've come under the shadow of a naysayer. One of those people who isn't rowing the boat, therefore they have plenty of time to rock it. They offer criticisms without offering help. They focus on something they don't like rather than seeing the vast amount of goodness they could like.

Yup, I suspect a naysayer has tried to pooh-pooh on you too. Especially during your healthy eating journey. But take heart, sweet sister, they are actually doing you a favor, if you'll let them. And I learned this in the strangest of ways.

I was recently in Virginia to appear on the *700 Club* when I got a frantic call from home. Apparently someone flushed too much toilet paper and caused a situation. An overflowage situation. You know it's not going to be a good call when you pick up the phone and hear your husband declare, "We are now a two-square family. No one in this house is allowed to use more than two squares of toilet paper at a time."

Oh my. That's hard for a girl, y'all. But it certainly was no time to argue with a man who was ankle deep in toilet water.

I love my man. Seriously, I do.

Apparently the water seeped down and around the caulking, into the walls, and onto the kitchen ceiling. Bummer.

The ceiling is now bulging and will most likely fall in. Lovely.

But we know some experts who can come in, cut out the sagging parts of the ceiling, patch it up, and put it all behind us.

And what, might you wonder, does this have to do with naysayers?

Here's the thing … had my husband known about the water coming out of the toilet early enough, he would have shut off the source to stop the unsightly flow.

As Jesus girls, we can't let the naysayers in life drown out our excitement, our commitment to healthy eating, and our assignments from Jesus. We have to shut off the source and stop the flow of negativity in our life.

We have to caulk up our cracks of insecurity with the putty of God's truth and assurance.

And we have an Expert who can cut out the sag in our hearts, patch it up with His sweet mercy, and put the whole thing behind us.

The naysayers want to distract us and knock us off course. But God says, "Stand firm. Let nothing move you. Always give yourselves fully to the work of the Lord, because you know that your labor in the Lord is not in vain" (1 Corinthians 15:58).

So, what favor do the naysayers do for us? They remind us we're doing something right for Jesus. I'd rather be criticized than ignored. I think Jesus would rather rein in wild Jesus girls kicking up some dust than kick dead-quiet mules any day of the week.

Whew, I love me some truth! Now, if I can just learn to love using only two squares of TP, all will be right with the world.

Dear Lord, please help me to cope with the difficult naysayers in my life. Show me Your truth to help me overcome the insecurities that follow me everywhere each day. Give me words, thoughts, and actions that honor and please You. Protect me from discouragement today. In Jesus' name. Amen.

Turning North

You have circled this mountain long enough.
Now turn north.
(DEUTERONOMY 2:3 NASB)

Thought for the Day:
Am I letting this mess *define* me or *refine* me?

We all have messes in our lives. We've been talking about the mess we can get into when we let our eating issues get out of control. But we face other types of messes as well. Financial messes. Relationship messes. Health messes. Kid messes. Home messes. Business messes.

Sometimes our messes are small and feel only like a slight annoyance. Other times, they're so huge they strip the hope right out of our lives. But here's a thought to ponder right in the midst of your mess ...

Am I letting this mess *define* me or *refine* me?

The answer to this question is crucial.

If I am letting a mess *define* me, I will feel *hopeless*.

If I am letting a mess *refine* me, I will be *hopeful.*

It's time for our messes to stop defining us.

It's time to embrace the refining process and "turn north."

If you find yourself stuck in a mess, try replacing your old self-defeating thoughts with empowering new thoughts. I call these "go-to scripts," statements of biblical truth that allow the Messiah to touch our mess and turn it into a great message of hope. Consider these:

1. *I was made for more than to be stuck in a vicious cycle of defeat.*

   "You have circled this mountain long enough. Now turn north" (Deuteronomy 2:3 NASB).

2. *When I am considering a compromise, I will think past this moment and ask myself, how will I feel about this choice tomorrow morning?*

   "Do you not know that your bodies are temples of the Holy Spirit, who is in you, whom you have received from God? You are not your own; you were bought at a price. Therefore honor God with your bodies" (1 Corinthians 6:19–20).

3. *When tempted, I will either remove the temptation or remove myself from the situation.*

   "God is faithful; he will not let you be tempted beyond what you can bear. But when you are tempted, he will also provide a way out so that you can endure it. Therefore, my dear friends, flee ..." (1 Corinthians 10:13b–14a).

4. *I don't have to worry about letting God down because I was never holding Him up; God's grace is sufficient.*

"But he said to me, 'My grace is sufficient for you, for my power is made perfect in weakness.'... For when I am weak, then I am strong'" (2 Corinthians 12:9–10).

5. *I have these boundaries in place not for restriction but rather to define the parameters of my freedom.*

"I put this in human terms because you are weak in your natural selves. Just as you used to offer the parts of your body in slavery to impurity and to ever-increasing wickedness, so now offer them in slavery to righteousness leading to holiness" (Romans 6:19 NIV 1984).

I keep these go-to scripts on the top of my mind so they interrupt the excuses I had become accustomed to believing for too long. Let some version of these statements bump into your reality and redefine your old patterns of thought. It will change the way you think!

And when we change the way we think, we'll be better equipped to change the way we make choices.

Dear Lord, help me to embrace and apply the truth in these go-to scripts. When I am weak, then I am strong. I want to leave my old eating habits behind me and turn this corner for good. In Jesus' name. Amen.

More than Feelings

Search me, God, and know my heart;
test me and know my anxious thoughts.
See if there is any offensive way in me,
and lead me in the way everlasting.

(PSALM 139:23–24)

Thought for the Day: We can't look to our feelings to determine truth. We must look to truth to rein in our feelings.

A few months ago I was speaking at a banquet where I met a precious young woman in her early twenties. She sheepishly made her way over to me with tears welling up in her eyes. She looked around before she whispered, "I don't feel saved. I have asked Jesus to be my Savior more times than I can count, but I just don't feel anything. What am I doing wrong?"

She wasn't doing anything wrong.

She was just looking in the wrong direction. She was looking for some magical feeling to swoop across the broken places of her life and instantly make everything feel different. That's not the way it works.

We can't look to our feelings to determine truth. We must look to truth to rein in our feelings.

Feelings are fickle. Feelings change on a whim. Feelings are paper thin and incapable of remaining untainted, unbiased, and unchanging. Faith can't be built on what we do or do not feel.

Truth, on the other hand, is stable, solid, and certain.

In the kindest way, I bossed her feelings with some truth. "You said you believe Jesus is the Savior, and you've confessed that with your mouth. You've asked Him to be the Lord of your life and for forgiveness of your sins. Right?"

She nodded, her eyes glistening with sincerity.

"Then park your mind, your heart, and your feelings on that truth and by the power of Jesus reject any lie that comes against that truth. You are saved. You are a child of God. You are eternally secure. Now, walk in that truth."

A wave of relief swept over her face. She threw her arms around me and buried her face in my jacket. I knew she was getting a little snot on my shoulder, and I could not have cared less.

I was too busy letting my own little sermonette make its way to my heart. I hadn't been doubting my salvation, but I had been doubting something else. I had been feeling afraid about releasing the message of *Made to Crave*.

After all, you can mess with a lot in a woman's life, but if you start messing with her food — that's grounds for serious irritation.

What if people didn't feel like embracing the message? What if people didn't feel like changing? What if it was just my issue and no one else really needed this message? What if people read it and remained unaffected and unchanged? What if I started backsliding in this area and made God look bad?

We can't look to our feelings to determine truth. We must look to truth to rein in our feelings.

I whispered these words over and over and over until they reached those raw places of insecurity deep in my soul.

Even if every single one of those feelings came to pass — people rejected the message and I gained my weight back — it wouldn't change or negate the absolute truths in the message. And it certainly wouldn't make God look bad. God doesn't build the stability of His identity on the fragile choices of His children. He just keeps placing the truth in front of us and offers to lead us to His best — over and over and over.

Dear Lord, I know I cannot look to my feelings to determine truth. I must look to You. Help me to be led by Your truth. Remove any doubts from my mind and lead me to freedom. In Jesus' name. Amen.

Accountability:
Helpful or Detrimental?

You will keep in perfect peace
those whose minds are steadfast,
because they trust in you.
(ISAIAH 26:3)

Thought for the Day: Whether accountability is positive or negative depends on where the conversations are focused. What we focus on becomes bigger and more magnified.

In the middle of a radio interview about *Made to Crave*, the show's host opened the phone lines for questions. Much to my surprise the first caller was a man. He was using the message of *Made to Crave* to overcome his struggles with pornography. He confessed that for years he'd tried to win this battle using an accountability partner.

It sounds good to have a friend who will hold you accountable. And it can be crucial.

But it can also be detrimental.

Whether accountability is positive or negative depends on

where the conversations are focused. What we focus on becomes bigger and more magnified.

The radio caller confessed that when meeting with his accountability partner, he'd make mental notes of all the inappropriate sites his accountability partner confessed during their time together — and then later visited those sites himself. Instead of helping his addiction, this accountability relationship actually fueled his failure.

It wasn't until the two men changed the focus of their conversations from porn to truth that they made progress. When the caller focused on the porn, his thoughts became more and more conformed to his pattern of sin. When he focused on truth, he became more and more transformed into a pure man of God.

Wow, did this make complete sense to me. My physical struggle is not the same as this man's struggle, but my physical struggle with food can be just as alluring and consuming. What might happen if instead of focusing our conversations on the scale, the food, and the hardship of sacrifice, we focused instead on asking each other questions about truths like these?

- *Our goal is letting the peace of God rule in us.* "You will keep in perfect peace those whose minds are steadfast, because they trust in you" (Isaiah 26:3). Are you at peace?

- *Our desire is to honor God with our bodies.* "Do you not know that your bodies are temples of the Holy Spirit, who is in you, whom you have received from God? You are not your own; you were bought at a price. Therefore honor God with your bodies" (1 Corinthians 6:19–20). How did you honor God with your body this week?

- *Our objective is to fill our soul with an abundance of truth instead of filling our stomach with an abundance of food.* "Then you will know the truth, and the truth will set you free" (John 8:32). What truths were you filled with this week?

Of course, part of accountability is to ask the tough questions about the physical struggles as well. But we shouldn't make this our focus.

If we want to grow closer to God, we have to distance ourselves from the distractions holding us back. And part of the distancing process is focusing on and magnifying God more and more … especially in our time of accountability.

Dear Lord, I truly understand how important good accountability is. As I progress through this journey, help me to continue to keep my focus on Your truth. Help me to focus on the things I can eat rather than the things I can't eat. I desire to honor You with my body, which is a temple of the Holy Spirit. Use me to help others who struggle as I do. In Jesus' name. Amen.

The Cost

... in order that Satan might not outwit us.
For we are not unaware of his schemes.
(2 CORINTHIANS 2:11)

Thought for the Day:
How much will this really cost me?

It is so crucial that we understand the fight we are in for our health, our families, our attitudes, our marriages, our friendships, our journey toward freedom. Satan wants not just to discourage us but to destroy us. His attacks are not just willy-nilly attempts to trip us up or knock us down. He wants to take us out.

I have a fire in my belly about how crafty and strategic Satan really is. He has made me fighting mad recently, and I can't help but address it.

Do you know why Satan's tactics are called schemes (2 Corinthians 2:10 – 11)? A scheme is a plan, design, or program of action. Satan's tactics are called schemes because they are well thought through plans specifically targeted to do three things:

1. To increase your desire for something outside the will of God.

2. To make you think giving in to a weakness is no big deal.

3. To minimize your ability to think through the consequences of falling to this temptation.

Oh how I wish we could see the cost of each of our choices as clearly as a price tag on store merchandise. Or as clearly as the caloric cost of food choices offered on menus in New York. (Did you know restaurants in New York are required to put nutritional information on their menus? Fabulous!) If I know how much something is going to cost me, I make much wiser choices.

Satan is a master of keeping that cost hidden until it's too late.

Here's how pastor and author Chip Ingram characterizes Satan's schemes:

> They are orchestrated in order to tempt us, deceive us, draw us away from God, fill our hearts with half-truths and untruths, and lure us into pursuing good things in the wrong way, at the wrong time, or with the wrong person. The English word *strategies* is derived from the Greek word Paul uses that is translated "schemes." That means our temptations are not random. The false perspectives we encounter do not come at us haphazardly. The lies we hear, the conflicts we have with others, the cravings that consume us when we are at our weakest points — they are all part of a plan to make us casualties in the invisible war. They are organized, below-the-belt assaults designed to neutralize the very people God has filled with his awesome power.[*]

Sweet sisters, I think this is something worth thinking about.

---

[*]Chip Ingram, *The Invisible War* (Grand Rapids: Baker, 2006), 27.

How much will this really cost me? If we do nothing else this week but consistently apply this one question to every choice, we will have invested wisely. So, so very wisely.

Dear Lord, please help me to focus on You today and the perfect plan You have for my life. I am reminded that boldly following You is so much better than any short-term experience that is not pleasing to You. Give me Your eyes so that I can see temptation and its many different faces. In Jesus' name. Amen.

Because Sometimes
I Want to Stop

LORD my God, I called to you for help,
and you healed me.
(PSALM 30:2)

Thought for the Day:
God is big enough to handle my doubts.

Before *Made to Crave* was published, I was working to develop a webcast to release at the same time as the book. Everything was cruising along when all of a sudden I hit an emotional brick wall.

Worry swept over me. My heart started beating fast. And suddenly, I wanted to stop the whole thing—the webcast, the book, the teaching videos, the workbook—all of it.

A voice that sounded like my own swirled in my mind: A woman and her struggle with food is a really sensitive issue. You are going to make some women mad. You can mess with a woman's pride, her spending issues, her anger, her insecurity, and her envy ... but the minute you mess with her food, it isn't going to be pretty.

I visualized really ugly emails from women angered by the *Made to Crave* message. And I started feeling afraid, accused, and tired. I wanted to crawl into my bed and hide in the safety of that quiet, private place.

But I was supposed to meet up with my friend Holly for our daily morning run in a few minutes. She'd start calling, and if I didn't answer, she'd come looking for me. And no one wants to find her friend snoring in bed at 11 a.m. (Yes, I snore, but that is a terrible subject for another day.)

Anyhow, back to my bout of complete dread on a morning that started so bright and cheery. What happened?

Diabolos. That's what happened. Some insecure thoughts dressed up as doubts came knocking on the door of my heart. Instead of turning them away with truth, I swung the door wide and allowed discouragement and defeat to march right in.

The accuser. The slanderer.

In Greek, his name is *Diabolos*. Some call him Satan. I call him the enemy whose main goal is to separate us from the truth. As I noted in an earlier devotion, his name literally means "the one who casts something between two to cause a separation."

Anytime we feel separated from truth — separated from God and our identity in Christ — you can bet Satan is having a field day tricking our feelings into this bad place. If he can get us to feel as if God is far away, then we're tempted to believe God really is far away. This is a lie.

When faced with a lie, we must boss our feelings around with the reality of truth.

The reality in my situation is that the message of *Made to Crave* is crucial. It's truth. Not my truth, but God's truth. This message has freed me in ways I never dreamed possible. And it will free other women too. God called me to write this truth. He came close and whispered this message into my heart. He was close then and no matter what I feel in this moment, He's close now.

Some of the truths in *Made to Crave* are hard. Like step-on-your-toes-and-make-your-lips-purse-together-in-frustration hard. But I didn't invent these hard Bible truths; God did. And wrapped throughout the harder truths is a grace that is tender, magnificent, and so very empowering. I reminded myself that God is big enough to handle my doubts.

So I dragged myself out of bed, drove to Holly's, and preached a little truth to myself the whole way. I quoted God's Word and sang praise songs all out of key and loud. And I let His absolute truth boss me and boss me and boss me.

I'll be honest, I was still scared. But I was a little less scared. And that was good.

I bet as you've been going through this journey, Satan has been trying to separate you from your real identity and truth as well. Instead of feeling victorious, you felt defeated. Instead of feeling steadfast, you felt shaky. Instead of feeling like a healthy lifestyle is doable, you wondered if you'd soon reverse your progress. Maybe you've even crawled into bed a time or two and pulled the covers way high.

Being uncertain and scared and riddled with doubt some days isn't a sign of bad things to come. It's actually quite the opposite. After all, if great things weren't on the horizon, I don't think the enemy would be so bent on attacking us. Think about it.

Today, try using a little truth to boss your feelings around. Remember, this whole healthy-eating journey is based on God's Word. Let's anchor ourselves in what God promises He'll do for us Jesus girls who've struggled with food: "They loathed all food and drew near the gates of death. Then they cried to the LORD in their trouble, and he saved them from their distress. He sent out his word and healed them" (Psalm 107:18–20a).

God sent forth His word and healed them. Healed them. And all my Jesus girls said, "Amen!"

Dear Lord, I know You are big enough to handle all of my doubts. By Your word You have healed me. Now, help me walk in the reality that I am anchored in Your promises. Forevermore. In Jesus' name. Amen.

Why Am I Scared
to Pray Boldly?

*The prayer of a righteous person
is powerful and effective.*

(JAMES 5:16B)

Thought for the Day: Prayer does make a difference — a life-changing, mind-blowing, earth-rattling difference. We don't need to know how. We don't need to know when. We just need to kneel confidently and know the tremors of a simple Jesus girl's prayers extend far wide and far high and far deep.

Have you ever caught yourself in this journey toward health being a little reserved in prayer? Me too. Especially when it comes to bold commitment prayers.

Prayers where I boldly commit this journey to God. Prayers where I commit to following through. Prayers where I declare the Scriptures we've been studying as promises I can live out. Prayers where I ask God to help hold me accountable.

It's not at all that I don't believe God can do anything. I absolutely do. I'm a wild-about-Jesus girl. Wild in my willingness. Wild in my obedience. Wild in my adventures with God.

My hesitation isn't rooted in any kind of doubt about God. It's more rooted in doubts about myself and a hyper awareness of my weaknesses.

Can you relate?

I so desperately want to stay in the absolute will of God that I sometimes find myself praying with clauses. Like, "God, I want to commit this journey to You, but I'm really scared I'm going to fail." I wonder why I don't just boldly pray, "God, I commit this journey to You. The whole thing. The times I'm successful and the times I need grace." And then stand confidently that my prayers were not in vain no matter what the outcome.

The reality is God wants me to boldly pray. I am convinced boldly praying changes me. It boots me out of that stale place of religious habit into authentic connection with God Himself.

Prayer opens my spiritual eyes to see things I can't see on my own. And I am convinced prayer changes circumstances. Prayers are powerful and effective if prayed from the position of a righteous heart (James 5:16).

Prayer does make a difference — a life-changing, mind-blowing, earth-rattling difference. We don't need to know how. We don't need to know when. We just need to kneel confidently and know the tremors of a simple Jesus girl's prayers extend far wide and far high and far deep.

Letting that absolute truth slosh over into my soul snuffs out the flickers of hesitation. It bends my stiff knees. And it ignites a fresh, bold, even wilder fire within me. Not bold as in bossy and demanding. But bold as in, *I love my Jesus with all my heart, so why would I offer anything less than an ignited prayer life?*

So let's ask God boldly for what we need in all aspects of our lives. Including this Made to Crave journey. Maybe especially for this ongoing Made to Crave journey. And then ask again. Not so that we can manipulate the movement of God. But rather so we can position our souls to really follow Jesus throughout this entire journey.

And with that, our devotions come to an end. But I can't think of a better place to leave you than tucked safely in the arms of a Jesus to whom we absolutely must boldly pray.

Dear Lord, I believe that You are the giver of life and Lord over all things. Help me to pray with a fresh new boldness today. I am convinced that prayers change me. I trust You and depend on You, Lord, and seek to follow You in every way. In Jesus' name. Amen.

Dear Friend . . .

You know how you feel when you've just spent time with a fun friend and you don't want it to end? Well, that's how I feel about our time together. I am so touched you spent a little slice of your life reading this *Made to Crave* title that I'd like to continue our conversation by tackling another important topic. Since *Made to Crave* was about what we put into our mouths, I thought it only fitting to now cover what comes out of our mouths.

My next book, *Unglued*, is about making wise choices in the midst of raw emotions. You know, those feelings you hide from those you want to impress but spew on those you love the most? Yes, let's go there. I need to go there. And since I only write messages I need myself, there is sure to be the same kind of gut-honest admissions and revelations you found me making here in *Made to Crave*.

We'll laugh together. Ponder together. Learn together. Have our toes stepped on together. And let Jesus mess with us in the best kind of way.

I can't wait. And just in case you can't wait either, here's chapter one of *Unglued* (beginning on page 191). With love,

Read an excerpt from *Unglued*. Coming August 2012!

CHAPTER 1

Invitation to Imperfect Progress

Emotions aren't bad. But try telling that to my brain, pulsing with the reality I should be sleeping at 2:08 a.m. instead of mentally beating myself up.

Why had I become completely unglued about bathroom towels? Towels, for heaven's sake. Towels!

The master bathroom is the preferred bathroom in our house. Although my three girls have their own bathroom upstairs, they much prefer our more spacious bathtub downstairs. As a result, our bath towels are frequently hijacked. I'll hop out of the tub and reach for the freshly laundered towel I hung on the rack the day before only to discover it isn't there. Ugh. So I wind up using a hand towel. (A hand towel. Can you feel my pain?) And while using said hand towel, I mutter under my breath, "I'm banning the girls from our bathroom." Then, of course, I never do anything to make the situation better and the same scene gets repeated time and time again.

I'd been dealing with the bath towel, or lack thereof, situation for quite a while. Then Art got involved. Up to this point, he had somehow managed to escape the woes of using a hand towel. But not this day. And his happiness did not abound upon discovering nothing but air where the towel should have been.

Since I happened to be nearby, he asked if I might please go get him a towel. I marched upstairs convinced I'd find every towel we own strewn randomly about my girls' rooms. I was preparing a little scolding speech as I went. With each step, I felt more and more stern. But when I went from room to room, there were no towels. None. How could this be?

Completely baffled, I checked in the laundry room. Nope, no towels there either. What in the world? Meanwhile, I felt the tension in my neck as Art called out once again.

"I'm coming, for heaven's sake," I snapped as I walked to the linen closet where the beach towels are kept.

"You'll just have to use one of these," I said as I tossed the large Barbie beach towel over the shower door.

"What?" he said. "Isn't this the towel the dogs sleep on?"

"Oh good gracious, it was clean and folded in the linen closet. I wouldn't give you a towel the dogs had been on!" Now my voice came out high-pitched and it was clear I was highly annoyed.

"Ugh. Is it too much to simply ask for a clean towel?" Art was asking a question, but to me it was more like a statement. A judgment. A slam against me.

"Why do you always do that?" I screamed. "You take simple mistakes and turn them into slams against me! Did I take the towels and hide them who-knows-where? *No!* Did I let the dog sleep on the Barbie towel? *No!* And furthermore, that isn't the Barbie towel the dogs were sleeping on. We have three Barbie towels — so there! Now you have the dadgum 4 – 1 – 1 on the towel issue. And none of this is my fault!"

I burst into tears and ran upstairs to give the girls a piece of my mind. "Never! Ever! Ever! You are *not* allowed to use the towels in our bathroom ever, ever, ever again! Do you understand me?"

My girls denied using the towels, which only made me madder. I punctuated each step I took heading back downstairs like a writer slamming her pen on the point of an exclamation mark.

Back downstairs, I grabbed my purse, slammed the door, and screeched the car tires on the driveway as I peeled off to a meeting. A meeting for which I was now late and in no mood to participate. It was probably some meeting about being kind to your family. I wouldn't know. My mind was a blur the rest of the day.

And now it's 2:08 a.m., and I can't sleep.

I'm sad because of the way I acted today. I'm disappointed in my lack of self-control. And the more I relive my towel tirade, the more my brain refuses sleep.

I have to figure this out. What is my problem? Why can't I seem to control my reactions? I stuff. I explode. And I don't know how to get a handle on this. But God help me if I don't get a handle on this. I will destroy the relationships I value most and weave my life with threads of anger, short-temperedness, shame, fear, and frustration. Is that really what I want? Do I want my headstone to read, "Well, on the days she was nice, she was really nice. But on the days she wasn't, rest assured, hell hath no fury like the woman that lies beneath the ground right here."

No. That's not what I want. Not at all. I don't want the script of my life to be written that way. So at 2:08 a.m., I vow to do better tomorrow. But better proves illusive and my vow wears thin in the face of annoyances and other unpleasant realities. Tears run down my cheek; I'm worn out from trying. Always trying.

So who says emotions aren't bad? I feel like mine are. I feel broken. Unglued, actually. I have vowed to do better at 2:08 a.m. and 8:14 a.m. and 3:37 p.m. and 9:49 p.m. and many other minutes in between. I know what it's like to praise God one minute and in the next minute yell and scream at my child — and then to feel both the burden of my destruction and the shame of my powerlessness to stop it.

I also know what it's like to be on the receiving end of this kind of unglued behavior, how painful it is to feel the sting of someone else spewing at me. The disrespect, the hurt, and feeling so misunderstood that I want to hurt the one who hurt me.

And the emotional demands keep on coming. The unrelenting insecurity. Wondering if anyone appreciates me. Feeling tired, stressed, and hormonal.

Feeling unglued is really all I've ever known. Maybe it's all I'll ever be?

Those were the defeating thoughts I couldn't escape. Maybe you can relate. If you relate to my hurt, I pray you also relate to my hope.

What kept me from making changes was the feeling I wouldn't do it perfectly. I knew I'd still mess up and the changes wouldn't come instantly. Sometimes we girls think if we don't make instant progress, then real change isn't coming. But that's not so. There is a beautiful reality called *imperfect change*. The day I realized the glorious hope of the imperfect change is the day I gave myself permission to believe I really could be different.

Imperfect changes are slow steps of progress wrapped in grace.

And good heavens, I'd need lots of that. So I dared to write in my journal:

> Progress. Just make progress. It's okay to have setbacks and do-overs. It's okay to draw a line in the sand and start over again — and again. Just make sure you're moving the line forward. Move forward. Take baby steps, but at least take steps that keep you from being stuck. Then change will come. And it will be good.

These honest words enabled me to begin rewriting my story. I couldn't erase what had come before, but I stopped rehashing it and turned the page afresh. Eventually, I started blogging about my raw emotions and imperfect changes. In response, I got comments whispering, "Me too."

"Being unglued, for me, comes from a combination of anger and fear," wrote Kathy. "I think part of it is learned behavior. This is how my father was." Theresa honestly admitted, "What makes me come unglued? Ignorance! Hatred! A non-forgiving spirit! Cruelty! A holier-than-thou attitude! Wow, I didn't know I had so many. I just walk around saying, 'Lord, help me!' That's all I can find to say." Oh, Theresa, I understand. Sometimes all I can think or say is, "Lord, help me."

And the comments kept coming, all of them expressing the exact same struggle, the same frustration, and the same need for hope. Women with kids and women without kids. Women caring for aging parents and women struggling with being the aging parent. Women working in the home and outside the home. So many different women whose daily circumstances differed but whose core issues were the same.

I realized then that maybe other women could make some imperfect progress too. And this book was born from that simple realization. But I had to laugh at the irony of it. I had just published a book called *Made to Crave* that dealt with what goes into my mouth. Now I was writing a book called *Unglued* to deal with what comes out of my mouth.

Unglued is about my imperfect progress — a rewrite for the ongoing script of my life and a do-over of sorts for my raw emotions. It's an honest admission that this struggle of reining in how I react has been hard for me. But hard doesn't mean impossible.

How hard something is often depends on your vantage point. Consider the shell of an egg. Looking at it from the outside, we know an eggshell is easily broken. But if you're looking at that same shell from the inside, it seems an impenetrable fortress. It's impossible for the raw white and tender yolk to penetrate the hardness of the eggshell. But given time and the proper incubation, the white and yolk develop into a new life that breaks through the shell and shakes itself free. And in the end, we can see that the hard work of cracking the shell was good for the baby chick. The shell provided a place for new life to grow, and then enabled the chick to break forth in strength.

Might the same be true for our hard places? Might all this struggle with our raw emotions and unglued feelings have the exact same potential for new life and new strength?

I think so. I know so. I've seen so.

Indeed, emotions aren't bad.

God gave us emotions. Emotions allow us to feel as we experience life. Because we feel, we connect. We share laughter and know the gift of empathy. We can drink deeply from love and treasure it as only emotions will allow. And yes, we also experience difficult emotions such as sadness, fear, shame, and anger. But might these be important as well? As being able to feel the hot stove tells our finger to pull back, might our raw emotions be important indicators as well?

Yes, but I must remember God gave me emotions so I could experience life, not destroy it. There is a gentle discipline to it all. One I'm learning.

So, in the midst of my struggle and from the deep places of my heart I scrawled out simple words about lessons learned, strategies discovered, Scriptures applied, imperfections understood, and grace embraced. I wrote about peace found, peace misplaced, flaws admitted, and forgiveness remembered. And eventually, I celebrated progress made.

And that's the promise of this book. Progress. Nothing more. Nothing less. We won't seek instant change or quick fixes. We'll seek progress. Progress that will last long after the last page is turned.

We will walk through our progress together. You're not alone. Neither am I. Isn't that good to know? Isn't it good to have this little space and time together where it's okay to be vulnerable with what we've stuffed and to be honest about what we've spewed?

There will be tender mercies for the raw emotions. No need to bend under the weight of past mistakes. That kind of bending breaks us. And there's already been enough brokenness here. No, we won't bend from the weight of our past, but we will bow to the one who holds out hope for a better future. It's a truth-filled future where God reveals how emotions can work for us instead of against us.

Our progress is birthed in this truth, wrapped in the understanding that our emotions can work for us instead of against us. And then we get to cultivate that progress, nurture it, and watch it grow. Eventually, others will begin to see it and take notice.

That's progress, lovely progress. Imperfect progress, but progress nonetheless.

Oh dear friend, there is a reason you are reading these words. There is a hurt we share. But might we also drink deeply from God's cup of hope and grace and peace as well? The fresh page is here for the turning. A new script is waiting to be written. And together we will be courageous women gathering up our unglued experiences and exchanging them for something new. New ways. New perspectives. New me. New you. And it will be good to make this imperfect progress together.

About Lysa TerKeurst

Lysa TerKeurst is a wife to Art and mom to five priority blessings named Jackson, Mark, Hope, Ashley, and Brooke. The author of more than a dozen books, including the *New York Times*-bestselling *Made to Crave*, she has been featured on *Focus on the Family*, *Good Morning America*, the *Oprah Winfrey Show*, and in *O Magazine*. Her greatest passion is inspiring women to say yes to God and take part in the awesome adventure He has designed every soul to live. While she is the cofounder of Proverbs 31 Ministries, to those who know her best she is simply a car-pooling mom who loves her family, loves Jesus passionately, and struggles like the rest of us with laundry, junk drawers, and cellulite.

> **WEBSITE:** If you enjoyed this book by Lysa, you'll love all the additional resources found at *www.MadetoCrave.org*.

> **BLOG:** Dialog with Lysa through her daily blog, see pictures of her family, and follow her speaking schedule. She'd love to meet you at an event in your area! *www.LysaTerKeurst.com*.

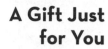

A Gift Just for You

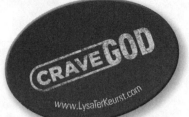

Get this free colorful magnet to keep you inspired and on track. The only charge is $1.00 for shipping and handling. Order by emailing: *Resources@Proverbs31.org* and put "Made to Crave Magnet" in the subject line. Bulk orders for Bible studies and small groups are also available with special shipping rates.

To download other free inspirational sayings, be sure to visit *www.MadetoCrave.org*, where you'll find many additional resources.

About Proverbs 31 Ministries

If you were inspired by *Made to Crave* and yearn to deepen your own personal relationship with Jesus Christ, I encourage you to connect with Proverbs 31 Ministries. Proverbs 31 Ministries exists to be a trusted friend who will take you by the hand and walk by your side, leading you one step closer to the heart of God through:

- *Encouragement for Today*, free online daily devotions
- The *P31 Woman* monthly magazine
- Daily radio program

To learn more about Proverbs 31 Ministries, contact Holly Good (*Holly@Proverbs31.org*), or visit *www.Proverbs31.org*.

Proverbs 31 Ministries
616-G Matthews-Mint Hill Road
Matthews, NC 28105
www.Proverbs31.org

Made to Crave

Satisfying Your Deepest Desire with God, Not Food

Lysa TerKeurst
President of Proverbs 31 Ministries

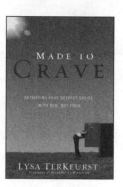

Made to Crave is the missing link between a woman's desire to be healthy and the spiritual empowerment necessary to make that happen. The reality is we were made to crave.

Craving isn't a bad thing.

But we must realize God created us to crave more of Him. Many of us have misplaced that craving by overindulging in physical pleasures instead of lasting spiritual satisfaction. If you are struggling with unhealthy eating habits, you can break the "I'll start again Monday" cycle, and start feeling good about yourself today. Learn to stop beating yourself up over the numbers on the scale. Discover that your weight loss struggle isn't a curse but rather a blessing in the making, and replace justifications that lead to diet failure with empowering go-to scripts that lead to victory. You can reach your healthy weight goal — and grow closer to God in the process.

This is not a how-to book. This is not the latest and greatest dieting plan. This book is the necessary companion for you to use alongside whatever healthy lifestyle plan you choose. This is a book and Bible study to help you find the want-to in making healthy lifestyle choices.

Available in stores and online!

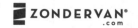

Made to Crave DVD Curriculum

Satisfying Your Deepest Desire with God, Not Food

Lysa TerKeurst
President of Proverbs 31 Ministries

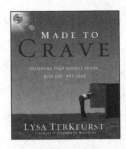

According to author Lysa TerKeurst, craving isn't a bad thing, but we must realize God created us to crave so we'd ultimately desire more of Him in our lives. Many of us have misplaced that craving, overindulging in physical pleasures instead of lasting spiritual satisfaction.

For a woman struggling with unhealthy eating habits, *Made to Crave* will equip her to:

- Break the "I'll start again Monday cycle" and start feeling good about herself today
- Stop beating herself up over the numbers on the scale and make peace with the body she's been given
- Discover how weight loss struggles aren't a curse but, rather, a blessing in the making
- Replace justifications that lead to diet failure with empowering go-to scripts that lead to victory
- Eat healthy without feeling deprived
- Reach a healthy weight goal while growing closer to God in the process

Made to Crave session titles include:

Session 1: From Deprivation to Empowerment

Session 2: From Desperation to Determination

Session 3: From Guilt to Peace

Session 4: From Triggers to Truth

Session 5: From Permissible to Beneficial

Session 6: From Consumed to Courageous

Bonus Session: Moving the Mountain

The *Made to Crave* DVD is designed for use with the *Made to Crave Participant's Guide*.

Made to Crave Action Plan Participant's Guide with DVD

Your Journey to Healthy Living

Lysa TerKeurst and Dr. Ski Chilton

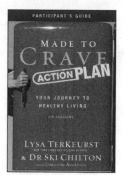

According to *New York Times* bestselling author Lysa TerKeurst, craving isn't a bad thing, but we must realize God created us to crave so we'd ultimately desire more of Him in our lives. Many of us have misplaced that craving, over-indulging in physical pleasures instead of lasting spiritual satisfaction.

Made to Crave Action Plan — a follow-up curriculum to *Made to Crave* — will help women implement a long-term plan of action for healthy living. In this six-session video-based study, women will be encouraged by Bible teaching from Lysa, uplifted by testimonies from women like Christian music chart-topper Mandisa, and empowered with healthy living tips from Dr. Ski Chilton, an expert in molecular medicine.

This curriculum will help women who found their "want to" by participating in the *Made to Crave* study master the "how to" of living a healthy physical life as well as cultivate a rich and full relationship with God. *Made to Crave Action Plan* gives women of all ages biblical encouragement for both their physical and spiritual journeys plus healthy living tips for use in their everyday lives.

Sessions include:

1. **Take Action:** Identify Your First Steps
2. **Eat Smart:** Add Fish and Increase Fiber
3. **Embrace the Equation:** Exercise and Reduce Calories
4. **Maximize Key Nutrients:** Increase Nutrient-Rich Fruits and Veggies
5. **Practice the Five Principles:** Keep Working Your Plan
6. **Make a Courageous Choice:** Direct Your Heart to Love and Perseverance

Becoming More Than a Good Bible Study Girl

Lysa TerKeurst
President of Proverbs 31 Ministries

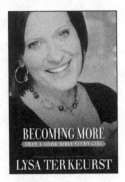

Is Something Missing in Your Life?

Lysa TerKeurst knows what it's like to consider God just another thing on her to-do list. For years she went through the motions of a Christian life: Go to church. Pray. Be nice.

Longing for a deeper connection between what she knew in her head and her everyday reality, she wanted to personally experience God's presence.

Drawing from her own remarkable story of step-by-step faith, Lysa invites you to uncover the spiritually exciting life we all yearn for. With her trademark wit and spiritual wisdom, Lysa will help you:

- Learn how to make a Bible passage come alive in your own devotion time.

- Replace doubt, regret, and envy with truth, confidence, and praise.

- Stop the unhealthy cycles of striving and truly learn to love who you are and what you've been given.

- Discover how to have inner peace and security in any situation.

- Sense God responding to your prayers.

The adventure God has in store for your life just might blow you away.

Available in stores and online!

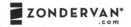

Becoming More Than a Good Bible Study Girl DVD Curriculum

Living the Faith after Bible Class Is Over

Lysa TerKeurst
President of Proverbs 31 Ministries

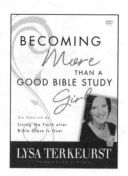

"I really want to know God, personally and intimately."

Those words of speaker, award-winning author, and popular blogger Lysa TerKeurst mirror the feelings of countless women. They're tired of just going through the motions of being a Christian: Go to church. Pray. Be nice. That spiritual to-do list just doesn't cut it. But what does? How can ordinary, busy moms, wives, and workers step out of the drudgery of religious duty to experience a living, moment-by-moment, deeply intimate relationship with God?

In six small group DVD sessions designed for use with the *Becoming More Than a Good Bible Study Girl Participant's Guide*, Lysa shows women how they can transform their walk with God from lackluster theory to vibrant reality. The *Becoming More Than a Bible Study Girl* DVD curriculum guides participants on an incredible, tremendously rewarding journey on which they will discover how to:

- Build personal, two-way conversations with God.
- Study the Bible and experience life-change for themselves.
- Cultivate greater authenticity and depth in their relationships.
- Make disappointments work for them, not against them.
- Find incredible joy as they live out their faith in everyday circumstances.

Available in stores and online!

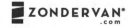

Share Your Thoughts

With the Author: Your comments will be forwarded to the author when you send them to *zauthor@zondervan.com*.

With Zondervan: Submit your review of this book by writing to *zreview@zondervan.com*.

Free Online Resources at
www.zondervan.com

Zondervan AuthorTracker: Be notified whenever your favorite authors publish new books, go on tour, or post an update about what's happening in their lives at www.zondervan.com/authortracker.

Daily Bible Verses and Devotions: Enrich your life with daily Bible verses or devotions that help you start every morning focused on God. Visit www.zondervan.com/newsletters.

Free Email Publications: Sign up for newsletters on Christian living, academic resources, church ministry, fiction, children's resources, and more. Visit www.zondervan.com/newsletters.

Zondervan Bible Search: Find and compare Bible passages in a variety of translations at www.zondervanbiblesearch.com.

Other Benefits: Register to receive online benefits like coupons and special offers, or to participate in research.

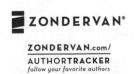

ZONDERVAN

ZONDERVAN.com/
AUTHORTRACKER
follow your favorite authors